HOME
MEDICAL
DICTIONARY

1992 Edition

P.S.I. & Associates, Inc.
13322 S.W. 128th Street
Miami, Florida 33186
305-255-7959
28397

Abacterial, sterile, free of bacteria.

Abalienation, mental derangement.

Abarognosis, loss of sense of weight.

Abarticular, not affecting a joint.

Abarticulation, dislocation.

Abasia, unable to walk because of loss of motor coordination.

Abatement, lessening of pain.

A.B.C. Process, purifying water or sewage by use of alum, blood and charcoal.

Abdomen, area of body between diaphragm and pelvic bones. The abdomen is lined with a smooth, transparent membrane called the peritoneum.

Abdominal, pertaining to the abdomen.

Abdominal Wall, the muscles in front of and along the sides of the abdomen.

Abduce, abduct.

Abduct, movement of an extremity away from the body or of a part from the middle of the whole.

Aberration, different from normal action.

Abevacuation, incomplete evacuation.

Abeyance, condition of suspended activity.

Abiology, study of nonliving things.

Abionarce, insanity due to infirmity.

Abiosis, absence of life.

Abirritant, soothing.

Ablactation, weaning.

Ablation, removal.

Ablepsia, blindness.

Ablucent, detergent.

Ablution, a washing.

Abnormal, not normal.

Aborad, away from the mouth.

Abortion, termination of pregnancy before the child is able to exist outside the womb. There are three types of abortions. An accidental abortion, usually referred to as a miscarriage, may be due to abnormalities of the egg

3

or infant, glandular or nutritional problems in the
mother, as well as other internal problems.
On the other hand, a therapeutic abortion is a deliberate step, taken for medical reasons, to stop a pregnancy.
Therapeutic abortions are generally performed when
the life or the health of the mother is threatened by the
pregnancy. In this type of abortion, the decision to end
the pregnancy is made and carried out by a doctor.
The third type of abortion, deliberate abortion, is performed when the mother decides that she does not
wish to continue the pregnancy.

Abrachia, congenital absence of arms.

Abrade, chafe, roughen.

Abrasion, any injury which rubs off the surface skin, leaving
a raw, bleeding surface.

Abreaction, a method employed in psychoanalysis to relieve a patient's feelings of guilt or hostility by reenact-
ing the experience which brought on the feelings.

Abscess, collection of pus enclosed anywhere in the body,
formed when foreign organisms destroy tissue.

Abscission, surgical removal of a growth.

Absorb, to seep in.

Abstract, to take away from.

Abtorsion, turning outward of both eyes.

Abuse, excessive use, or misuse. The term is frequently
used in connection with drugs, such as in "drug
abuse."

Abutment, anchorage tooth for a bridge.

Acampsia, rigidity of a part or limb.

Acapnia, decrease in carbon dioxide in the blood.

Acarbia, decrease of bicarbonate in the blood.

Acarid, tick, mite.

Acathexia, inability to retain bodily secretions.

Acceleration, increase the motion or speed.

Accident, unpleasant, unexpected happening leading to or
causing an injury or death.

Acclimatize, to get used to a climate.

Accommodation, adjustment.

Accouchement, act of being delivered.

Accoucheur, an obstetrician or person trained as a midwife.

Accretion, accumulation of matter at a part.

Acedia, mental depression.

Acephalous, headless.

Acescence, sour.

Acetabulum, hollow area in the hip bone in which thigh bone fits.

Acetarsone, a drug derivative of arsenic used in the treatment of amebiasis.

Acetate, salt of acetic acid.

Acetic, sour like venegar.

Acetone, a colorless, inflammable solvent.

Acetychlorine, hormone secreted by the nervous system.

Acetylcholine, an acid found in the body. It plays an important part in nerve impluse transmissions.

Achalasia, inability of certain hollow, muscular organs to contract.

Achilles Tendon, the tendon at the back of the heel. It connects the muscles of the calf to the heel bone.

Achlorhydria, inability of the stomach wall to manufacture hydrochloric acid.

Acholic, without bile.

Achondroplasia, form of dwarfism in which the trunk is of normal size, the limbs are too short.

Achor, small skin elevation on hairy parts of body.

Achoresis, diminution of the capacity of an organ.

Achroma, absence of color.

Achromyan, antibiotic.

Achylia, absence of chyle, an emulsion of fat globules formed in the intestine.

Acicular, needle-shaped.

Acid, a sour substance that combines with metals, releasing hydrogen.

Acid Burns, burns caused by acids. Acid burns should be washed immediately to remove the acid. Treatment then consists of applying a solution of sodium bicarbonate (baking soda) or some other mild alkali to neutralize any chemical which remains on the skin. (An exception is an acid burn from carbolic acid which should be treated by washing the skin with alcohol.) The affected area is then washed with fresh water and gently dried. At this point it is treated as though it were a true burn.

Acid-forming, applied to foods, which when digested, leave a residue that is acid.

Acidity, excess of the hydrochloric acid normally found in the stomach.

Acidosis, condition in some diseases which causes more acid in the blood than normal. Acidosis can be caused by disease of or failure of the lungs or kidneys (the two body organs which help regulate acids and bases). It can also be caused by dehydration (including severe diarrhea), diabetes, and acid poisoning.

Acid Poisoning, poisoning by acid taken by mouth. The antidote for acid poisoning is usually an alkali diluted in water which is swallowed to neutralize the acid.

Acme, crisis.

Acne, skin condition found usually in adolescents in which glands of skin become infected. It is characterized by comedos (blackheads) and small skin elevations (with or without pus). Acne is caused by excessive secretions of grease from the sebaceous glands. The grease dries and blocks pore opening (blackheads) and sometimes becomes infected (skin elevations with pus, usually referred to as pimples). Treatment of acne includes a diet low in greasy foods. The diet will often prohibit chocolates and carbonated beverages. The use of astringents can be helpful. Acne will normally subside in the late teens when puberty is completed.

Acneform, resembling acne.

Acoria, insatiable appetite.

Acousma, hearing imaginary sounds.

Acoustic, relating to sound or hearing.

Acquired, obtained after birth.

Acral, affecting the extremities.

Acrid, irritating.

Acro, a prefix used to denote the hands or feet.

Acroarthritis, arthritis of the extremities.

Acrodolichomelia, hands or feet which are abnormally long.

Acromegaly, gigantism; state of excessive growth of the body caused by overactivity of the pituitary gland.

Acromion, the highest and outermost extension of the shoulder.

Acronyx, ingrowing nail.

Acropathy, disease of the extremities.

Acrophobia, fear of great heights.

Acrosphacelus, gangrene of the fingers or toes.

Acrotism, pulse defect.

A. C. T. H., Adreno-Cortico-Tropic-Hormone; hormone that stimulates one part of the adrenal gland.

Actinic, applies to those rays of sunlight beyond the violet end of the spectrum, which produce chemical change.

Actinomycosis, disease of cattle that can be transmitted to man. It is caused by the microorganism *Actinomyces bovis*. The infection forms abscesses in the neck, chest, and abdomen. It is treated with antibiotics such as penicillin.

Acuity, sharpness, clearness.

Acupuncture, one of the methods of treatment used for a variety of conditions, diseases, and disorders. The treatment is based on inserting needles into various specified points on the body.

Acute, illness which had a sudden beginning, a short course and severe symptoms.

Acyesis, female sterility.

Addiction, the condition of being physically or psychologically dependent on some foreign matter.

Addiment, complement.

Addison's Disease, condition in which adrenal glands are underactive, characterized by a deficiency of blood sugar, low blood pressure, and low temperature.

Adduct, movement of an extremity toward the body or parts toward the midline of the body.

Adenalgia, pain in a gland.

Adenase, enzyme.

Adenitis, inflammation of a gland.

Adenoidectomy, surgical removal of the adenoids.

Adenoids, lymph glands in back of nasal passage which function to trap germs and debris.

Adenoma, tumor consisting of glandular material.

Adenopathy, any disease of the glands.

Adenosine Triphosphate, a compound found in muscles which is the storage place for extra muscular energy (abbreviated ATP).

Adhesions, abnormal growing together of tissue following injury or operation.

Adiaphanous, opaque.

Adicity, valance.

Adipose, fatty.

Adipose Tissue, fatty connective tissue found under the skin and surrounding various body organs.

Adiposity, obesity.

Adjuvant, an auxiliary agent or medication.

Adneural, toward a nerve.

Adnexa, appendages or accessory parts of an organ.

Adolescence, the period of life from the onset to the conclusion of puberty.

Adrenal Gland, small gland immediately above each of the two kidneys. Each gland is approximately the size of a pea. Each gland is made up of two distinct parts, and each part has different functions. The outer layer, or adrenal cortex, is essential to life and life processes; the inner part, or adrenal medulla, while important, is not essential.

Adrenalin, hormone secreted by the adrenal gland, with many properties.

Adrenocorticotropic Hormone, a hormone secreted by the anterior pituitary. Adrenocorticotropic hormone (abbreviated ACTH) stimulates the adrenal cortex of the adrenal glands to secrete hormones. ACTH has been synthesized and has been used to replace secreted ACTH. More frequently, however, it is used as a diagnostic tool.

Adtorsion, turning inward of both eyes.

Adult, fully developed.

Adventitious, accidental or acquired; pertaining to the tough outer coat of an organ or blood vessel; occurring in unusual places.

Aeration, the process of giving off carbon dioxide and taking on oxygen, which occurs to blood in the lungs.

Aeriform, gaseous.

Aerobic, a term applied to any living organism which can live in an oxygen atmosphere.

Aeropathy, decompression sickness.

Aerophagy, air-swallowing spasms.

Afebrile, without fever.

Affect, feeling, mood.

Afferent, conducting toward a center.

Affinity, attraction.

Afterbirth, material from womb after childbirth.

After-pains, the contractions of the uterus after delivery.

Agalactia, absence of milk secretion.

Agar, form of seaweed used in treating constipation.

Age-adjusted Death Rate, death rates that have been standardized by age for the purpose of making comparisons between different populations or within the same population at various intervals of time. Also called age-adjusted mortality rate.

Agenesia, sterility; imperfect development.

Agent, something which acts upon or against something else.

Age-specific Death Rate, the ratio of deaths in a specific age group to the population of the same age group during a given period of time, such as a year. It is calculated by dividing the deaths that occurred among the specific age group during the year, by the mid-year population in the same group of the same year.

Ageusia, lack of sense of taste.

Agglutination, the part of the healing process in which the wound closes by adhesion.

Aggregation, clumping together.

Aging, the process of growing old.
Everyone is subject to aging, starting from the moment of conception. Aging is part of the growing process. As the individual matures, there takes place a constant and simultaneous tearing down of old tissue and a building up of new tissue. In children, the building up process is more rapid than the tearing down process. When the child becomes an adult, the tearing down process begins to catch up with the building up process. Throughout an individual's lifetime, he is subject to this simultaneous dual process.

Agitation, restlessness; mental illness.

Aglutition, inability to swallow.

Aglycemia, lack of sugar in the blood.

Agnail, a hangnail.

Agnogenic, of unkown origin.

Agony, extreme pain.

Agorophobia, extreme fear of open places.

Ague, an old-fashioned name for malaria or other fevers.

Ahypnia, insomnia.

Aid, assistance given to a person in need of help.

AIDS (acquired immune deficiency syndrome), a fatal disease caused by a virus known as HTLV III OR HIV (human immunodeficiency virus). AIDS is primarily transmitted through sexual intercourse, but it can also be transmitted when contaminated blood comes in contact with a cut or break in the skin. The virus attacks certain types of white blood cells, leaving the body vulnerable to some kinds of infections and to cancers such as Kaposi's sarcoma. Symptoms include fever, drowsiness, skin infections, weight loss, swollen glands, weakness, headaches, and brown or purple nodules on the lower parts of the legs (Kaposi's sarcoma). A test is available to determine the presence of the virus before symptoms develop.

Air, the gaseous mixture which constitutes the atmosphere.

Air Embolism, the blockage of any blood vessel by a bubble of air.

Air-sickness, sickness caused by high altitudes and motion during air travel.

Airway, instrument used to keep breathing passages open.

Akalamathesia, inability to understand.

Alae Nasi, nostril openings.

Alalia, speech impairment.

Alastrim, variola minor, a mild type of smallpox.

Alba, white.

Albinism, absence of pigmentation.

Albino, lack of pigment in the skin. The lack of normal pigmentation causes the skin and hair to be white and the eyes to be pink. Albinos must be careful of the amount of sun to which they are exposed.

Albumen, protein.

Albuminuria, albumin in urine.

Alcohol, a colorless liquid which can be used as an astringent or antiseptic. One type of alcohol, ethyl alcohol, is the major ingredient in wines, beers, and distilled beverages. In this form, alcohol is a colorless inflammable liquid which has intoxicating effects.

Alcoholism, drunkenness, an addictive disease characterized by a craving for alcohol and its effect in relieving psychic and physical pain.

Aldosterone, a hormone secreted by the adrenal cortex of the adrenal glands which regulates the amount of salt that is excreted by the kidneys.

Alexia, unable to read.

Algesia, sensitivity to pain.

Algid, cold.

Algogenic, causing pain; lowering temperature.

Algophobia, extreme fear of pain.

Alienist, psychiatrist.

Alignment, the act of straightening or placing in a line a body part which is out of shape or place.

Alimentary, pertaining to nutrition.

Alimentary Canal, that part of the digestive system consisting of the esophagus, stomach, and intestines.

Alimentation, act of nutrition.

Alkali, a base substance. In the body, alkalis are balanced by acids. Alkalis will turn red litmus paper blue. Lye, ammonia, and potash are alkalis.

Alkalosis, an excess of alkaline in the body and bloodstream.

Allergen, that which produces an allergic reaction.

Allergist, specialist in allergies.

Allergy, abnormal sensitivity to any substance.

Allochroism, variation in color.

Allodromy, irregular heart rhythm.

Allopathy, the method of treating diseases and conditions by using drugs which produce effects opposite those from which the patient is suffering.

Aloe, vegetable used as a laxative.

Alogia, inability to form words; senseless behavior.

Alopecia, baldness.

Alveoli, tiny air sacs found at the end of bronchioles in the lung.

Alvine, pertaining to the belly.

Alzheimer's Disease, a rare disease in which there is mental deterioration similar to senility, but the disease occurs in middle age.

Amaurosis, blindness.

Ambidextrous, proficient with each hand.

Amblyacusia, dullness of hearing.

Amblyopia, dimness of vision due to errors of refraction.

Amblyopia Ex Anopsia, a condition of reduced or dim vision in an eye which appears to be normal. It sometimes is called "lazy eye." It occurs when the two eyes do not see the same thing with the same degree of clarity, and the poorer eye is not stimulated to develop or maintain clearness of vision. An example is when the eyes are not straight or have grossly unequal vision. Amblyopia ex anopsia usually is not caused by a disease process and it can generally be corrected if discovered early enough. The condition usually begins in children during pre-school years and may go undiagnosed into adulthood.

Ambulatory, able to walk.

Ambustion, burn, scald.

Ameba, a simple single cell protozoan.

Amebiasis, an infection of the bowel caused by a microscope ameba whose technical name is *Entamoeba hist olytica.* The infection can occur in mild or severe forms. In its severe form, amebiasis is known as amebic dysentery. More rarely, the infection may spread to the liver or other parts of the body.

Amenia, amenorrhea.

Amenorrhea, stoppage of normal menstrual periods.

Amentia, mental impairment.

Amine, an organic compound that may be derived from ammonia by the replacement of one or more of the hydrogen atoms by hydrocarbon radicals.

Amino Acids, a chemical radical in all proteins.

Ammonia, colorless gas which is soluble in water.

Amnesia, loss of memory.

Amniocentesis, procedure used to withdraw amniotic fluid from the uterus in order to ascertain if the baby has certain abnormalities.

Amniotic Fluid, the fluid in which the fetus lives until birth.

Amorphous, shapeless.

Amphetamines, drugs which stimulate the central nervous system. They induce a transient sense of well-being, self-confidence, and alertness.

Ampule, container for hypodermic solutions.

Ampulla, widened end of a small passageway.

Amputation, removal of a limb or appendage. The primary reasons for amputations are trauma, death of tissues due to inadequate circulation, malignant tumors, chronic infections of bone or tissue, heat or cold injuries, uselessness in a limb, and congenital deformities.

Amyasthenic, muscular weakness.

Amyl Nitrite, a drug that has the primary purpose of relaxing smooth muscles.

Amyloid, starchlike.

Amylophagia, eating of starch.

Amylopsin, an enzyme secreted from the pancreas. Amylopsin converts partially digested starches into simple sugars such as maltose.

Amylum, starch.

Amyotonia, flaccidity of muscles.

Amyotrophic Lateral Sclerosis, a disease causing paralysis because of degeneration of spinal cord.

Amyxia, absence of mucus.

Ana, of each.

Anabolism, any body process that builds complex compounds from simple compounds.

Anadipsia, intense thirst.

Anaerobic, a term applied to any living organism that cannot live in an oxygen atmosphere.

Anal, pertaining to the anus.

Analgesic, drug used to relieve pain.

Analygesia, lack of feeling any pain.

Analysand, one undergoing psychoanalysis.

Analysis, an examination of the different parts or elements that make up the whole.

Anamnesis, patient's history.

Anandria, absence of male characteristics.

Anaphase Stage, the stage in cell division (mitosis) during which the chromosomes are pulled or drawn toward the two poles. The anaphase stage follows the metaphase stage and precedes the telophase stage (the last step in cell division).

Anaplasia, a phenomenon of tumors (benign or malignant) in which the cells composing the tumor revert to simple, unspecific cells incapable of performing the highly developed, very specific functions associated with the tumor area.

Anemic, pertaining to anemia.

Anmeophobia, extreme fear of winds and draughts.

Anepia, inability to speak.

Anesthesia, loss of sensation.

Anesthesiology, study and administration of anesthetics.

Anesthetic, drug or gas used to abolish pain.

Aneuria, deficiency of nervous energy.

Anaphia, lack of sense of touch.

Anaphrodisia, loss of sexual desire.

Anastattis, highly astringent.

Anastole, retraction.

Anatomy, science which deals with the structure of the body.

Ancipital, two-edged.

Anconal, pertaining to the elbow.

Androcyte, spermatid.

Androgen, any substance or hormone causing masculine characteristics.

Androphobia, fear of men.

Androsterone, an important male sex hormone.

Anemia, condition in which the normal amount of red blood cells is reduced. Hemoglobin is the red-colored substance in the red blood cells; it carries oxygen to the body tissues. If the amount of hemoglobin is below normal, or if there are too few red blood cells, not enough oxygen will get to the tissues.

Anesthetics, substance that artifically produces complete or partial lack of feeling.

Aneurysm, swelling in a blood-vessel arising from the stretching of a weak place in the wall. Surgery on an aneurysm generally involves the removal of the aneurysm and the damaged areas around it. The length of artery or vein that is removed is replaced by a section of vein from another part of the patient's body or by a synthetic section of tube.

Anfractuous, convoluted.

Angina, a choking, suffocating sense of pain.

Angina Pectoris, severe attacks of pain over the heart. Angina pectoris is not a disease itself, but a symptom of a disease. Chest pains may be the result of many conditions other than an insufficient flow of blood to the heart muscle.
The symptoms appear with exertion, emotion, exposure to cold, or overeating, and can be relieved by rest or nitroglycerine.

Angiogram, an examination of a blood vessel by means of X-rays.

Angitis, inflammation of a vessel.

Anhelation, shortness of breath.

Anhematosis, defective blood formation.

Anhydrous, containing no water.

Anhypnosis, insomnia.

Aniline, a poisonous substance which is the base for both phenacetin and acetanilid, two drugs used as analgesics and antipyretics.

Anility, like an old woman.

Animation, liveliness.

Anisomastia, inequality of the breasts.

Ankle, region between the foot and lower leg.

Ankylosing Spondylitis, immobility of the vertebrae similar to rheumatoid arthritis.

Ankylosis, partial or complete rigidity of a joint produced either by disease, such as arthritis, or deliberately, by surgical operation.

Ankyroid, hooklike.

Annectent, connecting.

Annular, ring-shaped.

Annulus, circular opening.

Anodmia, absence of the sense of smell.

Anodyne, pain reliever.

Anoia, idiocy.

Anomaly, abnormality.

Anopheles, a genus of mosquitoes that transmits malaria to humans.

Anopsia, defective vision.

Anorchism, absence of testes.

Anorexia, loss of appetite. Anorexia can be caused by a nervous condition. It is more of a symptom than a disease. People with high fevers often exhibit anorexia. Certain drugs will also induce it. Among those are drugs prescribed as diet aids for people who are overweight.

Anoscope, instrument used for rectal examination.

Anoscopy, examination of the anus.

Anosmia, lack of sense of smell.

Anostosis, defective formation of bone.

Anoxemia, reduction in the normal amount of oxygen in the blood.

Anoxia, insufficient supply of oxygen. This condition most frequently occurs when the blood supply to a part of the body is completely cut off. This results in the death of the affected tissue.
However, anoxia may also occur when the entire body is lacking in oxygen as a result of breathing air with a low percentage of oxygen.

Ansa, looplike structure.

Antabuse, proprietary drug used in the treatment of alcoholism.

Antacid, substance that neutralizes acids.

Antebrachium, forearm.

Antemortem, before death.

Antenatal, before birth.

Ante-Partum, before maternal delivery.

Anterior, before.

Anteversion, forward displacement of part of the body, particularly the womb.

Anthelmintic, drugs used to rid the body of worms.

Anthophobia, extreme dislike of flowers.

Anthorisma, swelling.

Anthracosis, inflammation of the lungs due to inhalation of carbon dust.

Anthrax, disease of man from animals; two forms exist, one on skin and other in lungs.

Antianemic Principle, substance which counteracts anemia.

Antiarthritic, that which relieves or cures arthritis.

Antibechnic, relieving cough.

Antibiotics, the group of drugs usually prepared from molds or mold-like organisms, which are used in treatment of specific infections. Antibiotics are either bacteriostatic or bactericidal. That is, they inhibit growth of bacteria (bacteriostats) or they destroy them (bactericides). In either case, they work with the body's own defense system to cure the illness.

Despite the remarkable effectiveness of antibiotics against a wide range of diseases caused by bacteria, antibiotics do have drawbacks. Some people are hypesensitive, or allergic, to antibiotics.

The use of antibiotics may also lead to superinfections. These are infections caused by bacteria that normally live in the body without causing illness. The action of an antibiotic may upset the natural bacterial balance within the body, causing usually harmless bacteria to multiply into infections.

Antibody, a protein produced by body which reacts specifically with a foreign substance in the body.

Antibromic, deodorant.

Anticarcinogen, an environmental agent offering some protection against a carcinogen which is similar in chemical construction.

Anticoagulants, a group of drugs which reduce the clotting tendencies of the blood.

Anticus, anterior.

Antidote, remedy given to counteract a poison.

Antiemetic, remedy to prevent vomiting.

Antigen, any protein not normally present in the body and which stimulates the body to produce antibodies.

Antihemorragic, a general term for any drug or substance that helps slow, stop, or prevent hemorrhaging.

Antihistamine Drugs, a series of drugs used in the treatment of allergy.

Antihypertensive Agents, drugs that are used to lower blood pressure.

Antilemic, counteracting plague.

Antimetabolite, a substance closely similar to an essential cell-building material. An antimetabolite will tend to replace the essential material.

Antipathic, opposite in nature.

Antipathy, dislike.

Antipyretic, anything that reduces fever.

Antirabic, counteracting rabies.

Antiseptic, substance used to inhibit growth or destroy germs. Antiseptics are used on the skin only. They are similar to disinfectants in that both kill germs, but disinfectants are too strong to apply to the human body.

Antiserum, a serum that contains antibodies. It is obtained by withdrawing blood from an animal that has manufactured the antibodies as a result of exposure to antigens.

Anti-Toxin, substance manufactured by the blood, which specifically neutralizes the poison (toxin) given off by a particular germ.

Antitussive, any drug or agent which relieves or prevents coughing.

Antixerotic, preventing dryness.

Anton's Symptom, the failure or inability of a person who is blind to recognize or accept the fact of his blindness.

Antrum, space within a bone, usually that in the maxilla or upper jaw.

Anuria, absence of urine flow.

Anus, outlet of the bowel.

Anvil, the small bone located in the middle ear, situated between the stirrup and the hammer.

Anxietas, anxiety, worry.

Anxiety, a psychological term indicating uneasiness, apprehension, and similar emotions and feelings.

Aorta, main artery leaving the heart.

Aortic insufficiency, a condition in which there is an improper closing of the valve between the aorta and the lower left chamber of the heart. This allows a backflow of blood.

Aortitis, inflammation of the aorta.

Aortography, an examination by X-ray of the aorta and its main branches. This is made possible by the injection of a dye which is opaque to X-rays.

Apandria, dislike of men.

Apanthropy, dislike of human society.

Apathic, not having sensation.

Aperient, mild laxative.

Aperture, opening.

Apex, a term used to indicate the top or uppermost part of a body organ.

The blunt, rounded end of the heart, directed downward, forward, and to the left is also referred to as the apex.

Aphagia, inability to swallow.

Aphakia, absence of a lens behind the pupil of the eye.

Aphasia, inability to form words.

Aphephobia, fear of being touched.

Aphonia, inability to speak.

Aphrodisiac, drug which produces sexual excitement.

Aphtha, white spot.

Aphthous Stomatitis, a disease that causes recurring outbreaks of blister-like sores inside the mouth and on the lips. The sores are called canker sores.

Apnea, a momentary loss of the impulse to breathe.

Apogee, state of greatest severity of a disease.

Apomorphine, an opium derivative that causes nausea and vomiting very rapidly after it has been injected. The primary use for apomorphine is to induce vomiting when the patient has swallowed a poisonous substance. It has also been used to help alcoholics and drug abusers.

Apoplexy, condition which is the result of decreased blood flow to part of brain, also called stroke.

Apostasis, abscess.

Apothecary, druggist.

Appendage, outgrowth.

Appendectomy, surgical removal of the appendix.

Appendicitis, inflammation of the appendix.

Appendix, fingerlike projection from the large intestine with no known function.

Appestat, a part of the hypothalamus which regulates hunger.

Appetite, desire for food.

Applicator, instrument used to make local application of medicine.

Apprehension, a psychological term indicating a feeling of uneasiness about future events.

Approximal, close.

Apsithyria, a nonphysical condition in which the patient is unable to speak. Apsithyria is caused by hysteria.

Apsychia, unconsciousness.

Aptyalism, lack of saliva.

Aqueous, watery.

Arachnidism, condition resulting from spider bite.

Arachnoid, fine, thin tissue.

Arbor Urinae, a burning sensation experienced during urination.

ARC (AIDS-related complex), a condition in which some of the milder syptoms of AIDS are experienced.

Arcate, curved.

Archepyon, very thick pus.

Arenoid, like sand.

Areola, ring of color around a particular point, e.g., the nipple.

Argentic, containing silver.

Arhigosis, an inability to feel cold.

Ariboflavinosis, deficiency of riboflavin.

Arm, region from shoulder to below. The arm is composed of three large bones: the humerus, the ulna, and the radius. The humerus extends from the shoulder to the elbow, where it meets the ulna and the radius. The ulna and radius extend from the elbow to the wrist.

Armamentarium, doctor's entire equipment.

Armpit, the area under the arm where it joins the shoulder. The armpit is a small, hollow area. Its proper name is axilla.

Arrest, stopping; restraining.

Arrhenic, pertaining to arsenic.

Arrhythmia, disturbance of normal rhythm.

Arrowroot, nutrient starch.

Arsenic, poisonous chemical element.

Arteria, artery.

Arterial Blood, oxygenated blood. The blood is oxygenated in the lungs, then passes from the lungs to the left side of the heart via the pulmonary veins. It is then pumped by the left side of the heart into the arteries, which carry it to all parts of the body. Arterial blood is bright red in color.

Arteriole, smallest sized artery.

Arterioplasty, operation in which the artery is reconstructed.

Arteriosclerosis, condition in which arteries of body become thickened and inelastic. Every artery throughout the body is subject to hardening, but the most often and most seriously affected vessels are the largest arteries, such as the aorta, the coronary arteries, and the arteries that feed the brain and kidneys. Arteries may harden in one part of the body more rapidly then in other areas.

Arteriostenosis, constriction of an artery.

Arteristis, inflammation of an artery.

Artery, vessel which carries blood away from the heart. Blood moves through the arteries in spurts corresponding to the contractions of the heart muscle, which is forcing blood throughout the body.

Arthralgia, pain in a joint.

Arthrifuge, remedy for gout.

Arthritis, inflammation of one or more joints. The exact cause is unknown. There are two main theories: infection, and that the body's own defenses go awry and attack its own tissues. Emotional stress is believed to play an important role.

Arthrocace, ulceration of a joint.

Arthrodesis, a surgical procedure to put a joint in a fixed, rigid position.

Arthronosos, any joint disease.

Arthropathy, any joint disease.

Arthrophyma, joint swelling.

Arthroplasty, an operation upon a joint to make it function.

Arthrosclerosis, stiffening of the joints.

Articulation, enunciation of speech; a joint.

Artificial, not natural.

Artificial Respiration, the act of restoring breathing, the best method being mouth to mouth respiration. The standard methods of artificial respiration are the mouth-to-mouth method (with variations) and several manual methods (back-pressure, arm-lift; chest-pressure, arm-lift; back-pressure, hip-lift). Of these the mouth to mouth method is considered the best. Although first advocated for infants and children, it is now the recognized method of choice.

Asbestosis, lung disease occurring in those who inhale asbestos or asbestos-like material.

Ascariasis, invasion of the body by roundworms.

Ascending Paths, term used for the paths nerve impulses take on their way to the brain.

Ascites (Dropsy), an accumulation of body fluid in the abdomen.

Asepsis, absence of infected material or infection.

Asexual, without sex.

Asexualization, castration.

Asiderosis, iron deficiency.

Asitia, dislike of food.

Aspermatism, nonformation of sperm.

Asphyxia, stoppage of breathing due to obstruction of the air passages. Drowning, electric shock, and gas poisoning are the three most common accidents likely to result in asphyxiation. Asphyxiation also occurs from such accidents as choking, hanging, and burial in materials like grain, sand, or gravel. Excessive use of alcohol or drugs may also cause breathing to stop. Also, some illnesses, such as poliomyelitis (sometimes called polio or infantile paralysis), may result in asphyxiation.

Aspirator, instrument for withdrawing fluids by suction.

Aspirin, Acetylsalicylic acid, commonly used to relieve headache.

Assay, examine.

Asteroid, shaped like a star.

Asthenia, lack or loss of strength.

Asthma, condition of lungs characterized by decrease in diameter of some air passages. The asthma sufferer has periodic attacks of difficulty in breathing, which may be mild or severe.

Astigmatism, a defect of eyesight caused by uneven curvature of the outside membrane of the eye.

Astringent, that which causes contraction and stops discharges.

Asynergy, lack of coordination.

Atactitia, loss of the sense of touch.

Ataxia, loss of co-ordinated movement caused by disease of the nervous system.

Atelectasis, noninflation or incomplete inflation of a lung or lungs at birth, and, in adults, collapse of a lung.

Atheroma, hardening of the arteries.

Atherosclerosis, form of hardening of the arteries.

Athetoid, a type of cystic fibrosis in which the patient shows constant uncontrolled motion.

Athetosis, repetitive, involuntary, slow movements.

Athelete's Foot, fungus infection of the foot. The symptoms of infection are: itching, cracking or scaling of the skin, and sometimes small blisters that contain a watery fluid. If the disease continues without treatment, there can be large blisters and raw places on the skin.

Athrombia, defective blood clotting.

Atlas, topmost vertebra in the spinal column.

Atocia, sterility in the female.

Atomization, breaking up of a liquid into a fine spray.

Atony, lack of normal tone.

Atopy, allergy.

Atoxic, not poisonous.

Atresia, absence of a normal body opening.

Atrial Septum, the muscular wall that divides the left and right upper chambers of the heart which are called atria.

Atrophy, decrease in size of a normally developed organ or tissue.

Atrichia, absence of hair.

Attack, the onset of illness.

Attenuation, weakening, thinning.

Audiogenic seizure, an attack or seizure similar to an epileptic attack but brought on by auditory stimulation. The sound is usually a very high pitch.

Audiograph, graph showing acuteness of hearing.

Audiology, science of hearing.

Audiometer, instrument for measuring acuteness of hearing.

Audiophone, hearing aid.

Auditory Canal, the outer part of the ear.

Aura, sensations experienced before the onset of a disease or convulsion.

Aural, pertaining to the ear or hearing.

Aureomycin, antibiotic.

Auricle, the part of the ear that projects out from the head.

Auris, ear.

Aurotherapy, treatment with gold salts.

Auscultation, part of physical examination which uses detection of sounds in body by use of stethescope to aid diagnosis.

Autism, morbid concentration, a mental disorder which develops in childhood. The most striking symptom of the autistic child is his almost total withdrawal into himself. Ironically, autistic children often are very intelligent.

Autoclave, sterilizer.

Autodermic, a skin graft coming from the patient's own body.

Autodigestion, self-digestion.

Autoerotism, sexual stimulation of self.

Autogenuous, self, generated.

Autoimmunity, a condition in which the body has developed a sensitivity to some of its own tissues.

Autointoxication, poisoning by toxins formed within the body.

Autokinesis, voluntary motion.

Automatic, involuntary motion.

Autonomic, independent in action or function.

Autophobia, extreme fear of solitude.

Autopsy, examination of a body after death to discover the cause of death.

Autonomic Nervous System, part of the central nervous system which supplies the internal organs. It is divided into two parts: the sympathetic and the parasympathetic nervous systems.

Avitamic Acid, vitamin C; ascorbic acid.

Autotoxin, toxin formed in the body.

Auxesis, increase in size.

Avitaminosis, disease resulting from a vitamin deficiency.

Avulsion, tearing away of a part.

Axilla, armpit.

Axillary, pertaining to the armpit.

Axillary Nerve, nerve involved in shoulder movement and general sensations in the shoulder area. The axillary nerve used to be called the circumflex nerve.

Azoospermia, absence of sperm in the semen.

Azote, nitrogen.

Baby Blues, a feeling of depression and weepiness experienced by many new mothers. There are many reasons why a feeling of depression may occur. Physical changes within the mother's body may trigger and deepen feelings of depression. Because the mind and the body are so delicately meshed, any profound physical readjustment is bound to be reflected in feelings and thoughts. The hormones secreted during pregnancy are no longer needed, and the supply of available energy may not match the increased demands of the day—and night.

Baby Teeth, the first teeth, also called primary or milk teeth. The baby teeth are formed long before birth; the permanent teeth begin to form in the baby's jaw about the time he is born. At about six months of age (earlier in some children, later in others), the first baby teeth appear, usually the lower front ones. These are followed at more or less regular intervals by the upper front teeth, the back teeth, and the cuspids (called eye or canine teeth).

Bacca, berry.

Baccate, berry-shaped.

Bacillary, pertaining to bacillus bacteria.

Bacillemia, presence of bacilli in the blood.

Bacilliform, similar to a bacillus in shape.

Bacilluria, presence of bacilli in the urine.

Bacillus, pl., Bacilli, one of the major forms of bacteria.

Bacitracin, an antibiotic drug.

Back, posterior part of the body from the neck to the pelvic girdle.

Backache, pain in spine or adjacent areas.

Backflow, fluid moving in the opposite direction from the way it should be moving. A faulty or incompetent valve will allow blood to flow back in the wrong direction.

Bacteremia, bacteria in the blood.

Bacteria, microscopic organisms.

Bacterial Endocarditis, an inflammation of the inner layer of the heart caused by bacteria. The lining of the heart valves is most frequently affected. Bacterial endocarditis is commonly a complication of an infectious disease, an operation, or an injury.

Bactericide, that which destroys bacteria.

Bacteriostatic, a term applied to any drug or agent that inhibits the growth of bacteria. Different bacteriostats act against different bacteria.

Bacteriuria, bacteria in the urine.

Bagassosis, lung disease.

Bag of Waters, the sac of fluid in which an embryo floats. The fluid keeps the fetus evenly warm and acts as a shock absorber to protect it from jolts and bumps.

Balanitis, inflammation of the tip of the penis or clitoris.

Balanus, tip of the penis or clitoris.

Balbuties, stammering.

Baldness, lack of hair.

Ballistocardiogram, a tracing of the movements of the body caused by the beating of the heart.

Ballistophobia, extreme fear of missiles.

Ballooning, distention of a cavity.

Ballottement, rebound of a part when pressure is released.

Balm, soothing ointment.

Balsam, an aromatic resin.

Bandage, piece of gauze or other material for wrapping any part of the body.

Banti's Syndrome, an anomoly of the spleen.

Barber's Itch, infection of the beard area, also known as sycosis.

Barbital, a drug used to depress the central nervous system.

Barbiturates, drugs used as a hypnotic or sleep producer. Properly prescribed and taken as directed in small doses, they relieve tension and anxiety. In larger doses (three or four times as much) they produce drowsiness and sleep. They are also used medically for such psychosomatic conditions as high blood pressure, peptic ulcer, spastic colitis, and other psychophysiologic disorders.

Barium, a toxic metallic element.

Barium Sulfate, powder used in an emulsion which a patient drinks prior to X-rays of the stomach and intestines.

Barren, sterile.

Baryecois, deafness.

Basal Ganglia, part of the nervous system located in the brain. They play an important role in the transmission of impulses involved in voluntary muscular movement.

Basal Metabolism, the processes and/or measurement of vital cellular activity in the fasting and resting state based on oxygen usage.

Basedow's Disease, a goiter (thyroid enlargement) condition which includes a rapid pulse and nervous symptoms.

Baseplate, plastic material for making dental trial plates.

Basic, opposite of an acid; fundamental.

Basilic Vein, large vein on the inner side of the upper arm.

Bastard, one born of an unwed mother.

Bath, method of cleansing; therapeutic treatment.

Bathophoia, extreme fear of high objects.

Battarism, stuttering.

Beaker, glass with a wide mouth.

Bearing Down, the expulsive effort of a woman in the second stage of labor.

Beat, throb due to the contraction of the heart or passage of blood through a vessel.

Bedbug, an insect found in temperate and tropical climates. Bedbugs are usually flat and red. They live in houses, particularly in furniture and beds, and feed on human blood.

Bedsores, lesions over pressure areas on body of a bedridden patient.

Begma, cough.

Behavior, the observable activity of an individual.

Belch, escape of gas from the stomach through the mouth.

Belladonna, drug used to help spasmodic disorders.

Bell's Palsy, paralysis of the facial nerve; shown in weakness of one side of the face. The eye on the affected side will not close properly, and it becomes impossible to blow out the cheeks or whistle.

Belly, stomach.

Bemegride, a central nervous system stimulant which is used as a respiratory stimulant and as one of the antidotes for barbiturate poisoning.

Bends, decompression sickness.

Benign, non-repeating when referring to a disease.

Benignant, not recurrent.

Benzedrine, the proprietary name of a nervous stimulant.

Benzothiadiazine, a drug used to increase the output of urine by the kidney.

Beriberi, disease, uncommon in this country, caused by eating food deficient in vitamin B.

Beryllosis, inflammation of the lungs due to beryllium oxide dust.

Bestiality, intercourse with an animal.

Beta Rays, negatively charged particles emitted by radium.

Betalin S, synthetic vitamin B.

Bex, cough.

Bicameral, having two cavities.

Biceps, major muscle of the upper arm.

Bicarbonate, salt containing two parts carbonic acid and one part basic substance.

Bicellular, composed of two cells.

Biceps, any muscle that has two heads or branches.

Bicuspid, premolar tooth.

Bifocals, eyeglasses that serve the dual purpose of correcting both near and far vision.

Bifurcate, forked.

Bile, liver secretion.

Biliation, excretion of bile.

Biliousness, mild upset of the liver caused by dietary indiscretion.

Biliuria, bile in the urine.

Binaural Hearing-Aid System, a hearing-aid system consisting of two complete hearing aids—microphone, amplifier, and receiver—one for each ear. For some people, the binaural system increases the directional sense and helps to separate wanted sounds from unwanted background noise.

Binder, broad bandage used to encircle and support.

Biochemistry, chemistry of living things.

Biologicals, medical preparations used in the treatment or prevention of disease.

Biology, science of life and living things.

Biolytic, able to destroy life.

Bion, any living organism.

Biopsy, tissue taken from a living person for study.

Biostatics, vital statistics.

Biotomy, vivisection.

Bipara, woman who has had two labors.

Birth, process of being born.

Birth Canal, the canal a baby passes through during the birth process. The canal consists of the cervix, vagina, and vulva.

Birth Control, measures used to prevent pregnancy.

Birth Injury, any injury to an infant during the birth process.

Birth-Mark, blemish on skin of new born child, which is usually permanent.

Bisexual, both sexes in one person.

Bismuthosis, poisoning due to use of bismuth, a drug formerly used in the treatment of syphilis.

Bistoury, surgical knife.

Bite, cut with teeth; puncture by an insect.

Blackblood, impure blood.

Black Death, bubonic plague.

Black Lung Disease (pneumoconiosis), occupational disease caused by inhaling coal dust. Constant exposure over a long period of time irritates the lungs, causing scar tissue to develop.

Blackout, sudden temporary loss of sight and even consciousness.

Blackwater Fever, form of malaria.

Black Widow, poisonous spider.

Bladder, collecting pouch for urine from kidneys.

Bladder Control, the ability to control the urge to urinate. From birth on, the bladder empties automatically. To empty it is the natural thing to do. To hold back is somewhat harder and takes training. Most babies are not ready to master such delicate timing until long past one year of age.

Bland, soothing; mild

Blastocyte, a cell in an embryo. Blastocytes are nonspecific or primitive cells that later become more specific or differentiated.

Blastoma, tumor.

Blear-eye, chronic inflammation of margins of eyelids.

Bleb, blister.

Bleeder, one suffering from hemophilia; an inborn incurable disease in which severe bleeding follows even a slight cut.

Bleeding, emitting blood. The term bleeding is usually used to indicate bleeding from capillaries when blood trickles or oozes from a wound. The term hemorrhaging usually indicates bleeding from an artery or from a vein. The difference is one of degree—hemorrhaging is always serious, and if unchecked it is often fatal. Bleeding can result from a small cut or wound and will usually clot of its own accord.

Bleeding Time, time necessary for the natural stoppage of bleeding from a cut, about 3 minutes or less.

Blenna, mucus.

Blennagenic, producing mucus.

Blepharitis, inflammation of the eyelids shown by redness, crusting, swelling and infection of the eyelashes.

Blepharon, eyelid.

Blindness, inability to see; blindness can be partial or total. Visual impairment may result from one or more of the following: disease, defective functioning of the various parts of the eye, defects in the shape of the eye, congenital defects, irritation, injury, and accidents.

Blister, collection of fluid under the skin.

Bloated, swollen beyond normal size.

Block, an obstruction or blockage. The term is also used to refer to an anesthesia that goes deep into the tissues but is restricted in area.

Blood, fluid contained in arteries and veins of body that carries nutrients to and waste away from all tissues. Made up of cells and plasma.

Blood Bank, storing place for reserve blood.

Blood Clot, coagulated mass of blood.

Blood Count, a procedure that determines the number and type of red and white blood cells per cubic millimeter of blood.

Blood Groups, categories under which all human blood can be classified.

Bloodletting, a very old method for treating disease. It involved cutting the patient and allowing him to bleed. The idea was that the disease would leave the body with the escaping blood. It is used today in a very few cases of heart trouble to reduce the amount of blood and hence the amount of work the heart is required to do.

Bloodshot, locally congested with blood.

Blood-Pressure, this term refers to two different pressures in the blood system; the systolic pressure, which is that existing when the heart contracts and the diastolic pressure when the heart is in full relaxation.

Blood Transfusion, a technique for replacing a patient's lost, diseased, or ineffective blood with fresh blood from a healthy donor.

Blood Type, classification of blood into different groups.

Blood Vessels, vessels that carry blood throughout the body. There are three major blood-vessel types: arteries, capillaries, and veins.

Bloody Flux, dysentery.

Blotch, a spot, usually red or pink.

Blue Baby, child born with a blue color due usually to a heart defect.

Blue Ointment, mercurial ointment.

Blushing, rush of blood to the face.

Body, the physical man; trunk.

Body Cavities, thorax, abdomen, pelvis.

Boil, infection of the skin.

Bolus, round mass; pill; food prepared for swallowing by mastication.

Bone Grafting, transplanting a healthy bone to replace missing or defective bone.

Bonelet, small bone.

Bone Onlay, portion of transplanted bone placed across a break in a bone.

Bones, framework of body, composed of calcium and elastic tissue.

Bone Wax, material used to pack bone in order to stop bone bleeding.

Booster Inoculations, shots given at intervals to maintain a level of immunity.

Boric Acid, an antiseptic used on skin to help infections.

Boss, protuberance at one side of a bone.

Botulism, the most dangerous form of food poisoning; botulism is usually the result of eating contaminated foods from cans. The bacteria that cause botulism are anaerobic. This means that they grow only in an oxygen-free atmosphere. Therefore, canned foods provide an ideal growing place for them.

Bowel, intestine.

Bowleg, a leg that curves outward, usually below the knee.

Box Splint, used for fractures below the knee.

Brachium, arm.

Bradycardia, slow heart rate.

Braidism, hypnotism.

Brain, the primary nervous structure which sends out and receives stimulations to and from the rest of the body.

Brain Fever, meningitis.

Breakbone Fever, acute epidemic febrile disease.

Breast, front of the chest; mammary gland.

Breast-Feeding, feeding a newborn child with human milk from the mother's breast. It is probably the safest and most desirable way to nourish a child, because nobody has ever improved on the formula that the breast secretes to nourish the baby. However, breast-feeding should not be relied on exclusively for complete nutrition for much longer than the first four months of life.

Breath, air inhaled and exhaled in the respiratory process.

Breathe, to inhale and exhale air.

Breathing, act of taking in air to the body and exhaling carbon dioxide.

Breech Presentation, a baby born buttocks or feet first.

Bright's Disease, kidney disease.

Broad-Spectrum Antibiotic, any antibiotic that is effective against many different types of bacteria.

Bromides, salts of bromine.

Bromidrosis, offensive body odor.

Bromide, any salt containing bromine.

Bronchial Tubes, the large tubes (bronchi) that lead from the windpipe and carry the air that has been breathed in through the mouth and nose.

Bronchiectasis, state in which the lung tissue around the end of the breathing tubes becomes infected with the formation of sac-like cavities which fill with infectious material.

Bronchiole, smallest subdivision of the breathing tubes within the lung.

Bronchitis, inflammation of the windpipe which divides and subdivides into narrower tubes making up the network of air passages within the lungs.

Bronchorrhagia, hemorrhaging in the bronchial tubes.

Brown Mixture, cough syrup containing opium and licorice.

Brucella, type of bacillus.

Bruise, any injury to the surface of the body in which the skin is discolored but not broken.

Bubonic Plague, fatal infectious disease.

Bucca, mouth.

Bug, small insect.

Buggery, sexual relations through the anus.

Bulimia, an insatiable appetite.

Bulla, large blister.

Bunion, thickened area of skin on skin on lateral side of big toe.

Burn, an injury to the body caused by high temperature. Burns are classified in several ways: by the extent of the burned surface, by the depth of the burn, and by the cause of the burn. Of these, the extent of body surface burned is the most important factor in determining the seriousness of the burn and plays the greatest role in the patient's chances for survival.

Bursa, a sac like cavity usually found in or near joints.

Bursitis, inflammation of a bursa.

Buttocks, the rounded portion of the lower back which joins the thighs.

Buttonhole, straight cut through the wall of a cavity.

Bysma, plug; tampon.

Bythus, lower abdominal region.

Byssinosis, irritation of the air passages in the lung due to inhalation of cotton dust.

Cacation, defecation.

Cachet, capsule.

Cachexia, extreme wasting and weakness found in the later stages of a severe illness or starvation.

Cachinnation, hysterical laughter.

Cacomelia, deformity of a limb. Cacomelia is congenital.

Cadaver, corpse.

Caduceus, symbol of the medical, i.e., the wand of Hermes.

Caffeine, stimulant found mainly in coffee. It is used as a stimulant, a diuretic, and in the treatment of migraine headaches.

Cainotophobia, extreme fear of anything new.

Caisson Disease, occurs in workers, such as divers, who work under high atmospheric pressure, occurs when the pressure is reduced too rapidly, and the nitrogen in the blood escapes in the form of bubbles.

Calamine, pink substance composed of zinc and iron oxides, used in the form of lotion to soothe the skin.

Calcaneus, heel bone.

Calcareous, chalky; containing calcium.

Calcicosis, inflammation of the lungs due to marble dust.

Calcification, calcium deposits within the tissues of the body.

Calcinosis, calcium deposit in the skin and its underlying tissue.

Calcium, element which is the basis of limestone, important in body skeleton and function.

Calculus, stone-like mass which may form in the body under abnormal conditions.

Calf, the fleshy part of the back of the leg.

Calibrator, instrument for measuring openings.

Callous, any thickening of the skin formed on the site of continual irritation, usually on the feet or hands.

Callus, the new tissue formed at the site of fracture when a bone heals.

Calmant, Calmative, sedative.

Calomel, mercurous chloride; formerly used in the treatment of syphilis.

Calorie, measure of energy intake and output in the body.

Calvities, baldness.

Camphor, drug obtained from the camphor tree and used to stimulate the skin.

Camphorated, containing camphor.

Camphor Test, test for liver disease. When camphor is given orally, glycuronic acid will appear in the urine Absence of this reaction indicates a disease of the liver

Canal, passage, duct.

Cancer, any malignant tumor. Malignant tumors, such as cancer, always endanger life. They choke out normal tissue as they extend to adjacent tissue layers. They may also spread to other parts of the body. New growths thus related to the original tumor are called metastases. Cancerous cells can spread throughout the body via the blood and lymph systems.

Malignant tumors are divided into two main classes: carcinomas, which develop in the lining and covering tissues of organs; and sarcomas, which develop in the connective and supportive tissues of the body. Bone cancers are sarcomas.

Cancroid, like cancer; a tumor; type of skin cancer.

Cancrum Oris, gangrene of the mouth.

Canine Teeth, four teeth (upper and lower) between the incisors and molars.

Canker, type of mouth ulceration.

Cannabis, the dried, flowering tops of the hemp plant. Also called marihuana and hashish.

Capillary, smallest blood vessel. The capillaries serve as the crossing point between the small arteries (arterioles), which carry oxygenated blood from the heart, and the small veins (venules), which return blood to the heart. The walls of capillaries are semipermeable, allowing the interchange of water, salts, glucose, etc., between the blood and tissue fluid.

Capsule, tissue covering a part; soluble coating surrounding medication.

Caput, head.

Caput Succedaneum, edema or an abnormal collection of fluid in and under the scalp of a newborn baby.

Carbo, carbon, charcoal.

Carbohydrates, the scientific name for sugars, starches and cellulose.

Carbolic Acid, coal tar derivative used as an antiseptic and disinfectant.

Carbon, element which is the characteristic constituent of organic compounds.

Carbon Dioxide (CO_2), colorless, odorless gas used with oxygen to promote respiration.

Carbon-Dioxide Poisoning, a result of an increase in the percentage of carbon dioxide in the body over six per cent. This causes the rate of respiration to increase to the point where it can strain the heart, slow reflexes, and cause unconsciousness and death. In a healthy body this is uncommon, because the body will compensate by increasing the rate of depth of breathing.

Carbon Monoxide, A colorless, odorless, tasteless gas, which is produced as a result of incomplete combustion of organic material.

Carbuncle, large boil.

Carcinogenic, causing cancer.

Carcinoma, particular type of cancer.

Cardiac, concerning the heart.

Cardiac Arrest, total loss of heart function.

Cardiac Catheter, a diagnostic device for taking samples of blood, or pressure readings within the heart chambers, that might reveal defects in the heart.

Cardiac Failure, heart failure.

Cardiac Opening, the opening between the esophagus and the upper part of the stomach.

Cardiogram, record of changes in electrical energy of heart cycle.

Cardiograph, apparatus for making a graph of heart cycle.

Cardiology, medical specialty dealing with the heart.

Cardiospasm, contraction of the muscles controlling the inlet to the stomach.

Cardiovascular, pertaining to the heart and blood vessels.

Cardiovascular Disease, any disease that affect the heart and the blood vessels.

Caries, condition of decay, usually applied to decay of the teeth.

Carminative, drug to aid digestion and relieve flatulence, e.g., ginger, peppermint.

Carnal, pertaining to the flesh.

Carnal Knowledge, sexual knowledge.

Carnivorous, flesh-eating.

Carotene, a pigment (yellow or red in color) found in carrots, sweet potatoes, leafy vegetables, milk, and eggs. The body can convert it to vitamin A.

Carotid, major artery leading to the brain.

Carotid Gland, a small gland located between the internal and external carotid arteries.

Carpal, relating to the wrist.

Carpal Tunnel, the passage in the wrist for the median nerve and the flexor tendons in the wrist.

Carpus, wrist.

Carrier, one who harbors disease germs without suffering from the disease himself.

Car Sickness, illness due to motion of a car.

Cartilage, gristle; there are three types in the human body—hyaline, fibrocartilage, and elastic cartilage. Cartilage differs from bone in that it has no blood vessels. If it is cut or torn, the damage must be repaired surgically.

Cascara, a laxative.

Case, particular example.

Caseation, conversion of tissue into a cheese-like substance by certain diseases.

Casebook, Physician's record book.

Casein, protein product of milk.

Cast, mold to hold bone rigid and straight.

Castor Oil, old-fashioned purgative.

Castrate, to remove the testicles or ovaries.

Castration Complex, extreme fear of injury to the sex organs.

Casualty, accidental injury.

Catabolism, the breaking down of complex compounds into simpler ones.

Catalepsy, general name to describe various states marked by loss of power to move the muscles.

Catalyst, agent which influences a chemical reaction without taking part in it.

Cataplasm, a poultice, usually medicated.

Catamenia, onset of first menstrual period.

Cataract, clouding of the lens of the eye which prevents clear vision; not a film growing over the lens, but a change in the lens itself.

Catarrh, any illness which causes inflammation of membranes with a discharge of mucus.

Catatonia, type of schizophrenia characterized by immobility.

Catgut, sheep's intestine twisted for use as a surgical thread.

Catharsis, purging.

Cathartic, purgative.

Catheter, tube for passage through body channels, usually to evacuate fluids.

Cathexis, emotional energy attached to an object.

Catoptric Test, a test for cataracts made by observing reflections from the eye lens and cornea.

CAT SCAN (computerized axial tomography), type of diagnostic x-ray used to give a three-dimensional picture.

Caustic, irritating, burning.

Cautery, application of a burning agent to destroy tissue.

Cauterization, application of heat or burning chemicals to the surface of the body.

Cavity, hollow space.

Cecostomy, establishing an artificial opening into the large intestine near the appendix for evacuation.

Cecum, first part of the large intestine.

Celiac, pertaining to the abdominal region.

Cell, small cavity; a mass of protoplasm containing a nucleus.

Cell Membrane, the semipermeable wall surrounding an individual cell composed of protein and fat molecules that carefully regulate admission to the cell.

Cellular, composed of cells.

Cellular Tissue, loose connective tissue that has large interspaces and is found under the skin, peritoneum, etc.

Cellulitis, deep inflammation of the tissues just under the skin caused by infection with germs.

Central Nervous System, the part of the nervous system that includes the brain and the spinal cord.

Centrifuge, a machine that rotates at high speeds and is used to separate substances according to their densities.

Cephalalgia, headache.

Cephalic, pertaining to the head.

Cephalotractor, a forceps used by an obstetrician during delivery.

Cerebellum, small part of the nervous system, situated at the back of the brain, which is concerned with coordination of movements and bodily functions such as respiration.

Cerebral Palsy, a broad term used to describe a variety of chronic conditions in which brain damage, usually occurring at birth, impairs motor function and control.

Cerebration, mental activity.

Cerebrospinal Fever, an acute infectious form of meningitis, also referred to as epidemic cerebrospinal meningitis. In addition to inflammation of the membranes of the brain and spinal cord, there is usually an eruption of hemorrhage spots on the skin.

Cerebro-Spinal Fluid, the clear fluid which surrounds the brain and spinal cord as they lie inside the skull and in the canal of the spinal column; acts mainly as a shock absorber.

Cerebrum, the brain, especially the large frontal portion, as distinct from the cerebellum and the spinal cord.

Cerumen, ear wax.

Cervical, pertaining to the neck or mouth of womb.

Cervix, the neck or that part of an organ resembling the neck.

Cervix Uteri, the narrow lower portion of the uterus.

Cesarean Operation, abdominal operation to remove a child from the womb of a pregnant woman.

Cestoid, resembling a tapeworm.

Chafing, irritation caused by the rubbing together.

Chalazion, tumor of the eyelid.

Chancre, the name given to the sore that appears on the body when infected with certain types of venereal disease organisms.

Chancroid, an infection of the genitals that is caused by *Haemophilus ducreyi.* The original sore is at the site of infection and can be quite painful. The infection can spread to the lymph nodes of the genital area. It is treated with sulphonamide drugs and sometimes with tetracycline.

Change of Life, the menopause, usually occurring in women between the ages of forty and fifty-five, and about ten years later in men.

Charcoal, a black carbon that results from the burning (or charring) of organic material.

Charley Horse, bruised or torn muscle associated with cramping pain in the muscle.

Charting, recording the progress of a disease.

Check, slow down; stop, verify.

Cheek, side of the face below the eye.

Cheilitis, inflammation of the lips.

Cheilosis, lip disorder due to vitamin deficiency.

Chemical Burn, a burn caused by acids, alkalies, or other chemicals.

Chemotherapy, the treatment of disease by chemicals or drugs.

Chest, area enclosed by the ribs and sternum.

Cheyne-Stokes Respiration, breathing that is characterized by changing depths of respiration.

Chicken Pox, relatively mild childhood disease. It is spread by secretions from the mouth and nose and by fluid from the characteristic skin blisters. The incubation period is two to three weeks.

Chilblains, painful swelling of fingers, toes and ears caused by exposure to cold.

Child, one in the period between infancy and youth.

Child Abuse, the willful injury of a child by parents or guardians.

Chill, symptoms that occur when one first becomes infected with any germs which cause fever; result of nervous stimulation.

Chin, area below lower lip.

Chiropractic, system of treatment based on the belief that all disease is caused by pressure on the nerves as they leave the spinal column.

Chiropractor, one who specializes in bone manipulation.

Chlamydia, venereal disease.

Chloasma, brownish discoloration of the skin found in patches on any part of the body; particularly apparent in some pregnant women.

Chloral Hydrate, a drug used as an hypnotic. It works as a depressant to the central nervous system. For a while the use of chloral hydrate was replaced by the barbiturates, but recently it has been used more frequently. It has a strong odor and a bitter taste and should not be taken on an empty stomach. Chloral hydrate is one of the drugs prescribed for insomnia.

Chloremia, decrease of hemoglobin and red corpuscles of the blood.

Chlorine, a yellow-green poisonous gas used in compounds as a disinfectant and antiseptic.

Chloroform, heavy, clear, colorless liquid used as an anesthetic.

Chloromycetin, antibiotic.

Chloroquine, a compound drug used in the treatment of malaria.

Chlorosis, form of anemia.

Chlorothlozide, a chemical compound that increases the output of urine.

Choke, obstruction of the pharynx or esophagus.

Cholecystis, the gallbladder.

Cholecystectomy, removal of the gall bladder.

Cholecystitis, inflammation of the gall bladder.

Cholelith, gallstone.

Cholemia, presence of bile in the blood.

Cholera, tropical intestinal disease.

Choleric, irritable.

Cholesterol, substance found in fats and oils.

Cholestasis, a condition in which the flow of bile from the liver is stopped or suppressed.

Cholinesterase, an enzyme.

Chondral, pertaining to cartilage.

Chondro, a prefix meaning cartilage.

Chondroma, a benign tumor containing the structural elements of cartilage.

Chopart's Amputation, an amputation of part of the foot.

Chorda, string, tendon.

Chordae Tendineae, fibrous chords that serve as guy ropes to hold the valves between the upper and lower chambers of the heart secure when forced closed by pressure of blood in the lower chambers.

Chorea, also known as St. Vitus' dance or Sydenham's chorea; disease of the nervous system, usually considered to be related to rheumatism or rheumatic fever.

Choriomeningitis, inflammation of the coverings of the brain.

Chorion, outermost of the fetal membranes.

Chorlocarcinoma, a cancer occurring in a part of the placenta sometimes retained in the uterus following pregnancy.

Chromatelopsia, color blindness.

Chromatic, pertaining to color.

Chromatid, one of the pair of spirals of a chromosome.

Chromatosis, pigmentation.

Chromocyte, colored cell.

Chromosome, one of several small more or less rod-shaped bodies in the nucleus of a cell.

Chronic, of long duration.

Chronological, according to time sequence.

Chrysoderma, a pigmentation of the skin resulting from deposits of gold.

Chylomicron, a minute particle of fat that is found in the blood during digestion.

Chyme, food after digestion in the stomach.

Cicatrix, scar.

Cilia, microscopic waving hairs.

Ciliary Muscle, the muscle that surrounds the eye lens and helps the eye to focus by changing the shape of the lens.

Circulation, flowing in a circular course.

Circulation Time, rate of blood flow.

Circulatory System, the system that consists of the heart, the arteries, the veins, and the capillaries.

Circumcision, operation of cutting off the foreskin of male penis.

Circumflex, a term used to denote a part of the body that winds around or bends around another part of the body.

Cirrhosis, hardening of any tissue, but particularly of the liver.

Cirsectomy, removal of a part of a varicose vein.

Citric Acid, a mild acid found in citric fruits such as lemons and grapefruit. It plays an important role in metabolism.

Clamp, surgical device for compressing a part or structure.

Claudication, lameness due to decreased blood flow.

Claustrophobia, extreme fear of enclosed spaces.

Clavicle, collar bone.

Clavus, corn.

Cleavage, division into distinct parts.

Cleft, fissure.

Cleft Palate, congenital fissure of the palate forming one cavity for the nose and throat.

Climacteric, change of life.

Clinic, bedside examination; center where patients are treated by a group of physicians practicing together.

Climax, period of greatest intensity.

Clinical, pertaining to bedside treatment.

Clinotherapy, treatment of a patient's complaints by bed rest.

Clitoris, small erectile organ of the female genitalia.

Clomiphene, a drug used to increase fertility.

Clot, to coagulate.

Clubbed Fingers, fingers with a short, broad tip and over-hanging nail, somewhat resembling a drumstick.

Club-Foot, congenital deformity of the feet of unknown cause.

Clunis, buttock.

Clyster, enema.

Coagulation, formation of a blood clot.

Coaguloviscosimeter, an instrument that measures the amount of time the blood takes to coagulate.

Coalescence, fusion of parts.

Coarctation, narrowing or constricting.

Cocaine, a highly addictive drug of abuse; a local anesthetic.

Cocci, a type of bacteria that are spherical in shape. "Cocci" is used as a suffix for denoting specific bacteria.

Coccygodynia, pain in the area of the tail bone.

Coccyx, small bones at the end of the spine.

Cochlea, cavity in the internal ear.

Codeine, sedative.

Cod-Liver Oil, the chief outside source of vitamins A and D, obtained from oil of cod fish.

Cognition, processes involved in knowing.

Coitus, sexual intercourse.

Coitus Interruptus, a method of contraception in which the penis is withdrawn before semen is ejaculated.

Colchicine, drug which helps to relieve symptoms of gout.

Cold Abscess, an abscess that develops slowly and shows little sign of inflammation. A cold abscess is generally tuberculous.

Colds, common viral infection of man causing symptoms of nasal fullness, cough and fever.

Cold Sores, lesions particularly in and around mouth caused by herpes simplex virus.

Colectomy, removal of part of the large intestine.

Colic, severe abdominal pain caused by spasm of one of the internal organs, usually the intestines; pertaining to the colon or large intestine.

Colitis, inflammation of the large intestine.

Collapse, to flatten; breakdown; prostration.

Collateral, a secondary or alternative path for the flow of blood.

Colles' Fracture, a fracture of the lower end of the radius.

Collodion, drug which, when painted on the skin, forms a thin transparent protective film.

Collyrium, local eye medication, e.g., eye wash.

Coloboma, a defect. Usually used to indicate a congenital defect of the eye.

Colon, large intestine.

Color Blindness, an inborn condition in which, while ordinary vision remains normal the individual is unable to distinguish between particular colors.

Colostomy, a surgical procedure that reroutes the colon to bypass and avoid the rectum.

Colostrum, first milk from a mother's breast after childbirth.

Colpalgia, vaginal pain.

Colpatitis, vaginal inflammation.

Column, supporting part.

Coma, complete loss of consciousness, which may be the result of various causes.

Comatose, state of being in a coma.

Comedo, blackheads in glands of skin.

Commensal, a term used to denote an organism that lives on or within another organism without causing harm to the host.

Comminute, a bone shattered in several pieces.

Comminution, breaking into small fragments.

Commissurotomy, an operation to widen the opening in a heart valve that has become narrowed by scar tissue.

Commitment, placing a patient in an institution.

Common Cold, a viral infection of the throat and nasal passages.

Comparative Anatomy, human anatomy compared to that of animals.

Compensation, a change made by the body to compensate for some abnormality.

Complication, added difficulty.

Compound, substance composed of different elements.

Compound Fracture, a fracture of the bone in which the broken bone pierces the skin.

Compress, a pad for application of pressure or medication to a specific area.

Conception, fertilization of an ovum by a sperm forming a zygote or fertilized egg which develops into an embryo.

Concha, shell-like organ.

Concussion, stunning; condition of dizziness, mental confusion and sometimes unconsciousness, due to a blow on the head.

Condom, rubber covering worn over the penis to prevent conception.

Conduction, conveyance of energy.

Condyle, the rounded protuberance at the end of a bone.

Condyloma, wartlike growth near the anus or genitals.

Congenital, existing at or before birth.

Congenital Heart Defects, a defect existing at birth, resulting from the failure of an infant's heart or of a major blood vessel near the heart to develop normally during pregnancy.

Congestion, excess accumulation of blood or mucus in any part of the body.

Conjunctiva, the membrane lining of the eyelid and outer surface of the exposed portion of the eyeball.

Conjunctivitis, inflammation of the transparent membrane which covers the eyeball.

Connective, that which binds together.

Connective Tissue, one of the four main tissues of the body which support bodily structures, bind parts together and take part in other bodily functions.

Consciousness, awareness.

Constipation, failure of bowels to excrete residue at proper intervals.

Constrictive Pericarditis, a shrinking and thickening of the outer sac of the heart, which prevents the heart muscle from expanding and contracting normally.

Consumption, tuberculosis.

Contact Lenses, a substitute for or an alternative to wearing eyeglasses. Contact lenses are usually round disks, concave in shape, to fit on the convex surface of the eyeball. The disk floats on the fluid of the eye and serves the same purpose as the lenses from a pair of eyeglasses—helping to adjust impaired vision.

Contagion, (see infection.)

Contagious, easily transmitted by contact.

Contagium, agent causing infection.

Contaminate, to soil or infect.

Continence, ability to control natural impulses.

Contraception, use of mechanical devices or medicines to prevent conception.

Contractile Protein, the protein substance within the heart muscle fibers responsible for heart contraction by shortening the muscle fibers.

Contraction, a drawing together.

Contracture, a shortening of tissue, causing deformity or distortion, e.g., scar.

Contraindication, a condition or factor that indicates that a particular treatment or drug is unsuitable for use in a specific case.

Contusion, bruise.

Convalescense, the period following an injury, illness, surgery, etc., during which the patient is recuperating.

Convex, rounded and somewhat elevated.

Convolutions, curved and winding inward folds, such as the surface of the cerebrum or the intestines.

Convulsant, medicine which causes convulsions.

Convulsion, temporary loss of consciousness with severe muscle contractions due to many causes; fit or generalized spasm.

Copulation, sexual intercourse.

Cord, Spinal, that portion of the central nervous system contained in the spinal canal.

Cord, Umbilical, cord which connects the umbilicus of the fetus to the placenta.

Corium, layer of skin under the epidermis.

Corn, thickening of the skin, hard or soft, according to location on the foot.

Cornea, transparent membrane covering the eye and lying beneath the conjunctiva.

Corneum, outermost layer of skin.

Coronary Artery Bypass, major heart surgery which removes one or more veins from the leg and uses them to bypass blocked arteries in the heart.

Coronary Atherosclerosis, an irregular thickening of the inner layer of the walls of the coronary arteries.

Coronary Thrombosis, clotting of blood in the blood vessels which supply the heart.

Coroner, one who holds inquests over those dead from violent or unknown causes.

Cor Pulmonale, heart disease resulting from disease of the lungs or the blood vessels in the lungs.

Corpus, principal part of an organ; mass.

Corpuscle, blood cell.

Corpus Luteum, a yellow substance secreted by the ovary after an ovum has been released.

Corrosive, destructive; disintegrating.

Corsucation, sensation of flashes of light before the eyes.

Cortex, outer layer of the brain and other organs.

Corticosteroids, hormones secreted in the adrenal cortex.

Cortisone, a hormone produced by the adrenal glands.

Costae, the twenty-four bones (twelve on each side) that form the rib cage.

Costalgia, rib pains.

Couching, a technique used in the treatment of cataracts. Instead of stripping the lens from the eye, the surgeon displaces or moves the cataract into a position where it cannot block light rays.

Cough, an attempt on the part of the body to expel something causing irritation in the respiratory tract.

Coumarin, a class of chemical substances that delay clotting of the blood. An anticoagulant.

Counterirritation, the application of an irritant to reduce or relieve another irritation. Counterirritation can involve the use of drugs in the form of ointments or the use of heat. Counterirritants are usually applied to the skin and seem to work by producing an inflammation, thus increasing the flow of blood to the affected area.

CPR (cardiopulmonary resuscitation), type of artificial respiration which maintains heart and lungs until professional help is available.

Cradle Cap, an accumulation of a thick, greasy crust, usually on the scalp; but it may occur behind the ears, on the eyebrows or eyelashes, at the corners of the nose, on the cheeks, or even on the truck.

Cramp, painful, spasmodic contraction.

Cranial Nerves, twelve pairs of nerves directly connected to the brain.

Cranium, skull.

Creatine, a compound of nitrogen manufactured in the body.

Cremaster, muscle which draws up the testis.

Crest, ridge on a bone.

Cretinism, condition caused by the lack of or decreased secretion of the thyroid gland in a child.

Crevice, small fissure.

Cricoid Cartilage, cartilage that forms the lower and back sections of the larynx.

Crisis, the turning point of a disease.

Critical, dangerous; severe.

Crohn's Disease, chronic inflammation of the intestinal tract.

Cross-eyes, condition in which eyes do not move together.

Cross Matching, a method used to be sure that the recipient and the donor involved in a blood transfusion are compatible blood types.

Croup, a disease of children characterized by coughing and difficult breathing.

-cule, -cle (suffix), little.

Cubitus, the elbow; also the forearm and hand.

Culture, propagation of an organism.

Cure, system of treatment; restoration to health.

Cusp, point of the crown of a tooth; pointed projection on a segment of a cardiac valve.

Cuspid, canine tooth.

Cut, a wound in which the skin is broken by a sharp cutting instrument or by material.

Cuticle, outermost layer of the skin.

Cutis, the outer layers of skin, including the epidermis and the dermis (or corium).

Cyanide, one of the fastest-acting poisons.

Cyanosis, term used to describe blueness of the skin, generally caused by lack of oxygen.

Cyclarthrodial, a term applied to any joint that can rotate.

Cyclomethycaine, a chemical preparation used as a local or surface anesthesia.

Cyesis, pregnancy.

Cyst, any sac in the body filled with liquid or semi-liquid substance.

Cystic Fibrosis, an inherited disease of children and adolescents that affects the exocrine, or externally secreting, glands of the body.

Cystitis, inflammation of the bladder.

Cystoscope, a lighted tube used in the examination of the urinary bladder.

Cystoscopy, process of examining the inside of the bladder with an instrument.

Cytochrome, a group of compounds found in animal and human tissues; they play an important role in the movement of oxygen from the blood to the cells.

— D —

Dacryorrhea, excessive flow of tears.

Dactyl, digit.

Dactylion, webbing of the fingers and toes.

Dactylitis, inflammation of a finger or toe.

Dactylology, communication with the fingers, i.e., sign language.

Dactylus, finger; toe.

Daltonism, color blindness.

D. & C., dilation and curettage of uterus.

Dandruff, condition of the scalp characterized by dry scaling.

Dapsone, one of the sulfone class of drugs used in the treatment of leprosy.

Dartos, fibrous layer under the skin of the scrotum.

Deaf-mutism, inability to hear or speak.

Deafness, complete or partial loss of hearing.

Dealbation, bleaching.

Dearterialization, conversion of arterial into venous blood.

Death Rate, number of people who die each year, compared with the total number of population.

Death Rattle, gurgling noise caused by passage of air through accumulated fluid in the windpipe.

Debility, weakness.

Decalcification, decrease in the normal mineral salts content of bone.

Decalvant, making bald.

Decerebration, removal of the brain.

Decidua, membranous lining of the uterus shed after childbirth or at menstruation.

Decompensation, failure of an organ to adjust itself to changing condition.

Decompression, removal of pressure.

Decompression Sickness, a condition caused by a rapid decrease in atmospheric pressure brought on by an excess of nitrogen in the blood and body tissues.

Decripitude, senile feebleness.

Decubitus, lying down posture.

Decubation, period of convalescence from an infectious disease.

Defecation, evacuation of the bowels.

Defective, imperfect.

Defemination, loss of female and assumption of male sex characteristics.

Defibrillator, any agent or measure that stops irregular contractions of the heart muscle and restores a normal heartbeat.

Deficiency Disease, any disease caused by the lack of some essential part of the diet.

Defloration, loss in a woman of virginal characteristics, i.e., rupture of the hymen.

Defluvium, falling out of hair.

Deformity, distortion, malformation.

Degeneration, deterioration or breaking down of a part of the body.

Deglutition, act of swallowing.

Dehydration, loss of water.

Dejecta, excrement.

Dejection, melancholy.

Delactation, weaning, stopping of lactation.

Deliquesence, liquefaction of a salt by absorption of moisture from the air.

Delirium, mental disturbance, usually occurring in the course of some infectious disease, or under the influence of poisonous drugs.

Deliver, to aid in birth.

Deltoid, triangular.

Delusion, false belief.

Demented, insane.

Dementia, deterioration of intelligence.

Dementia Praecox, the old term for schizophrenia.

Demorphinization, treatment of morphine addiction by gradual withdrawal.

Demulcent, reducing irritation; a soothing substance.

Dengue, tropical disease carried by mosquitoes, causing fever and joint pain.

Denigration, process of becoming black.

Dens, tooth.

Dentagra, toothache; forceps for pulling teeth.

Dental Caries, tooth decay. Three conditions are necessary for tooth decay. One is a susceptible individual, which includes nearly every American. This susceptibility may be related in part to hardness and other qualities of the enamel and dentin, which may influence resistance to decay. Another condition is the presence of decay-producing bacteria found in plaques, which are allowed to remain on the teeth. Equally important is a caries-producing diet with large amounts of carbohydrates, particularly sugar, taken into the mouth frequently.

Dentalgia, toothache.

Dentifrice, any substance used for cleaning teeth.

Dentin, chief substance of teeth.

Dentistry, branch of medicine dealing with teeth.

Denture, complete unit of teeth.

Deodorant, that which destroys odors.

Deontology, medical ethics.

Deorsum, downward.

Depersonalization, loss of the sense of one's own reality.

Depilate, to remove hair.

Depilatory, substance used to remove hairs.

Deplete, to empty.

Depraved, perverted.

Depressant, that which retards any function.

Depression, a feeling of melancholy, hopelessness, and dejection.

Derangement, disorder.

Dermad, toward the skin.

Dermatitis, inflammation of the skin, eczema.

Dermatologist, skin specialist.

Dermatology, branch of medicine which deals with the skin and its diseases.

Dermatosis, any skin disease.

Dermis, the true skin.

Dermoid, resembling skin.

Desensitization, a series of injections given to a patient who has an allergy.

Desiccant, a drying medicine; tendency to cause drying.

Desiccate, to dry.

Desmalgia, pain in a ligament.

Desquamation, the shedding of skin.

Detergent, cleansing.

Deterioration, the process of losing ground, or of getting worse.

Deviation, variation from the normal condition.

Dexter, right.

Dextrocardia, position of the heart in the right side of the chest.

Dextrophobia, extreme fear of objects on the right side of the body.

Dextrose, form of sugar.

Diabetes, a disease which shows itself in an inability of the body to handle glucose.

Diabetes Mellitus, a disorder of carbohydrate metabolism characterized by excessive sugar in the blood and urine and associated with a disturbance of the normal insulin mechanism.

Diagnosis, determination of a patient's disease.

Diagnostician, one skilled in determining the nature of a disease.

Di- (prefix, two.

Dialysis, a method of separating substances in solution form.

Diaphragm, large muscle which separates the inside of the chest from the inside of the abdomen; contraceptive device.

Diaphysis, shaft of a long bone.

Diarrhea, watery, loose bowel movements.

Diarticular, pertaining to two joints.

Diastole, period of relaxation of the heart during which it fills with blood.

Diastalsis, forward movement of the bowel contents.

Diastema, space, cleft.

Diathermy, treatment of disease or injury by use of heat.

Diathesis, type of constitution which makes one liable to a particular disease.

Dichotomy, division into two separate parts.

Dick Test, test to discover whether a patient is liable to or immune from scarlet fever.

Didymalgia, pain in a testis.

Diet, nutritional intake; prescription of food permitted to be eaten by a patient.

Dietetics, science of diet and nutrition.

Dietitian, specialist of diet in health and disease.

Dietotherapy, use of a diet regimen for cure.

Differentiation, a process of growth in the embryo from very general cells to very specific cells.

Diffuse, widely spread.

Digestant, that which aids digestion.

Digestion, assimilation of food by the body.

Digestive Tract, the system responsible for the body's breakdown and use of food. It is composed of the mouth, pharynx, esophagus, stomach, small intestine, large intestine (including the colon and rectum), and accessory glands.

Digit, finger; toe.

Digitalis, drug used in the treatment of heart diseases.

Dilatation, stretching; increase in diameter.

Dimercaprol, a heavy metal antagonist. Drugs such as dimercaprol are used as antidotes to heavy metal poisoning. Dimercaprol is effective against metals such as mercury and arsenic.

Dionism, homosexuality.

Diphasic, having two phases.

Diphtheria, disease causing the development of membrane in nose and throat.

Diploplia, double vision.

Dipsomania, excessive desire for drink.

Disarticulation, separation of bones at a joint.

Disc, Disk, platelike structure or organ.

Discharge, setting free; excretion.

Discipline, a body of knowledge or field of study with distinctive rules and assumptions.

Discrete, separate.

Disease, sickness; ailment.

Disengagement, liberation of the fetus from the vaginal canal.

Disinfectant, a fluid used to kill bacteria and other microorganisms.

Disinfectation, extermination of pests.

Disinfection, killing germs by antiseptics or other methods.

Disks, the pads (made of cartilage) that are located between each of the vertebrae.

Dislocation, displacement of the bones in a joint. Dislocations result from force applied at or near the joints, from sudden muscular contractions, from twisting strains on joint ligaments, or from falls where the force of landing is transferred to a joint. The joints most frequently dislocated are those of the shoulder, hip, finger, and jaw.

Dismemberment, amputation.

Dispensary, place which gives free or low cost medical treatment.

Displacement, a condition in which a body part has been moved out of its normal position.

Dissection, cutting up.

Disseminated Sclerosis, disease of the nervous system in which small patches of hard tissue (sclerosis) develop throughout the spinal cord and brain.

Distal, remote or removed from. The opposite of proximal.

Distention, widening; enlargement.

Distillation, purification of a liquid by vaporizing it and then condensing it.

Distrix, the splitting of the hairs at the end.

Diuresis, frequent urination.

Diuretic, medicine which increases the flow of urine.

Divagation, unintelligible speech.

Diverticulitis, inflammation of small pouches or diverticuli in large intestine.

Dizziness, sensation of spinning or off balance.

DNA, the abbreviation for deoxyribonucleic acid. DNA is one of the two nucleic acids found in all cells. (The other is RNA—ribonucleic acid.)

Dolorific, causing pain.

Domatophobia, extreme fear of being in a house.

Dominant Trait, a trait that can be inherited from only one parent.

Donor, one who gives blood or body tissue for the use of others.

Dope, a slang term applied to narcotic drugs when they are misused.

Doraphobia, extreme fear of fur.

Dorsal, pertaining to the back or hind part of an organ.

Dorsalgia, pain in the back.

Dorsum, back.

Dose, amount of medication to be given at one time.

Dose, Lethal, dose large enough to cause death.

Dossier, file containing a patient's case history.

Double-Blind, an experiment in which neither the patient nor the attending physician knows whether the patient is getting one or another drug.

Douche, stream of water directed into a body cavity or against the body itself.

Dowel, pin used to hold an artificial crown to a natural tooth root.

Down's Syndrome, a form of mental retardation. Also known as mongolism.

D.P.H., Department of Public Health.

DPT and Polio Injection, a shot given to develop immunity to diphtheria, pertussis (whooping cough), tetanus (lockjaw), and polio (infantile paralysis).

Dragee, large, sugar-coated pill.

Drain, channel of exit for discharge from a wound.

Drainage, a rubber tube inserted in the body, which allows excess fluid or pus to escape instead of collecting.

Dramamine, drug commonly used for seasickness.

Dreams, flowing images that occur during sleep.

Dressing, protective covering placed over a wound to aid the healing process.

Drive, basic urge.

Drop Foot, state of inability to raise the foot upwards due to paralysis of the leg muscles.

Dropper, tube for giving liquid in drops.

Dropsy, generalized accumulation of fluid in body, edema.

Drowning, suffocation and death due to filling the lungs with liquid.

Drug, any medicinal substance.

Drug Abuse, the deliberate act of taking a drug for other than its intended purpose, and in a manner that can result in damage to the person's health or his ability to function.

Drug Addiction, physical dependence on a drug. The definition includes the development of tolerance and withdrawal.

Duct, tube or channel that conducts fluid, especially the secretion of a gland.

Ductus Arteriosus, the passageway between the two major blood vessels that adjoin the heart: the aorta and the pulmonary artery.

Dumb, unable to speak.

Duodenum, first eight to ten inches of the small intestine.

Dura Mater, outermost covering of the brain and spinal cord.

Dwarf, an undersized person.

Dynamia, energy.

Dys- (prefix), bad; difficult.

Dysarthria, stammering.

Dysarthrosis, dislocation; disease or deformity of a joint.

Dysbasis, difficulty in walking.

Dyschiza, painful bowel movement.

Dysemesia, painful vomiting.

Dysentery, name given to a group of disorders in which there is diarrhea, produced by irritation of the bowels.

Dysfunction, impairment of function.

Dysgenesis, malformation.

Dysgraphia, inability to write.

Dyskinesia, impairment of the ability to make any physical motion.

Dysmenorrhea, painful menstruation.

Dyspepsia, indigestion.

Dyspnea, labored breathing.

Dystithia, difficulty in breast feeding.

Dystocia, difficult childbirth.

Dystrophy, weakening of muscle due to abnormal development.

Dysuria, painful urination.

Ear, organ of hearing. Consists of three different sections: the outer ear, the middle ear, and the inner ear.

Earache, pain in ear usually due to inflammation.

Eat, to take solid food.

Ebullition, boiling.

Eburnation, hardening of teeth or bone.

Ecbolic, that which speeds up child birth or produces abortion.

Eccentric, peripheral, peculiar in ideas.

Ecchymosis, a discoloring of the skin caused by the seepage of blood beneath skin.

Eccysesis, extrauterine pregnancy.

Ecdemic, pertains to disease brought into a region from without.

Echinococcosis, infestation with a type of tapeworm.

Echo, reverberating sound.

Echolalia, senseless repetition of words spoken by others.

Eclampsia, form of internal poisoning and convulsions which may occur in late pregnancy.

Ecouvillonage, cleansing of a wound or cavity.

Ecphuma, outgrowth.

Ecphyadectomy, appendectomy.

Ecstasy, exaltation.

Ectal, external.

Ectasia, widening in diameter of a tubular vessel.

Ecthyma, inflammation of the skin, characterized by large pimples that rupture and become crusted.

Ecthyreosis, absence of or loss of function of the thyroid gland.

Ectocardia, displacement of the heart.

Ectoderm, outermost layer of cells in a developing embryo.

-ectomy (suffix), excision.

Ectopic, abnormal position of an organ, part of a body; pregnancy outside the uterus.

Ectropion, the turning out of a part, particularly an eyelid.

Eczema, an itching disease of the skin.

Edema, an excessive accumulation of tissue fluid.

Edentate, without teeth.

Edeology, study of the genitalia.

Edible, suitable to be eaten.

Effemination, assumption of feminine qualities in a man.

Efferent, conducting away from a center.

Effluvium, foul exhalation.

Effort Syndrome, a group of symptoms (quick fatigue, rapid heartbeat, sighing breaths, dizziness) that do not result from disease of organs or tissues and that are out of proportion to the amount of energy that is used.

Effusion, accumulation of fluid, or the fluid itself, in various spaces of the body, e.g., joints.

Egesta, body excretions or discharges.

Egg, ovum.

Ego, that part of the mind which possesses reality and attempts to bring harmony between the instincts and reality.

Egocentric, self-centered.

Egomania, morbid self-esteem.

Egotism, exaggerated evaluation of one's self.

Eiloid, coiled.

Ejaculation, ejection of semen.

Ejaculum Praecox, premature ejaculation in the male.

Ejection, the act of expelling.

Elastic, able to return to normal shape after distortion.

Elation, joyful emotion.

Elbow, juncture at which the arm and forearm meet.

Electric Cardiac Pacemaker, an electric device that can control the beating of the heart by a rhythmic discharge of electrical impulses.

Electric Shock, shock caused by electricity. Electricity causes shock by paralyzing the nerve centers that control breathing or by stopping the regular beat of the heart.
The symptoms of electric shock are sudden loss of consciousness, absence of respiration (which, if present, is slight and cannot be detected), weak pulse, and probable burns. Every second of delay in removing a person from contact with an electric current lessens the chance of resuscitating him. It is important to act quickly, but the rescuer must be careful not to come in contact with the current or a conductor.

Electricity, form of energy having magnetic, chemical and thermal effects.

Electrocardiogram, a graphic record of the electric currents produced by the heart.

Electrocardiography, a machine which records the electrical activity of the heart muscles.

Electrocoagulation, the deterioration or hardening of tissues by high-frequency currents.

Electroconvulsive Therapy, a method of treating certain types of mental illnesses. Electroconvulsive therapy (ECT) involves passing an electric current or shock through the patient's brain.

Electrode, an electric conductor through which current enters or leaves a cell, an apparatus or body.

Electroencepalogram, record of the electrical changes of the brain.

Electrolyte, any substance that, in solution, is capable of conducting electricity by means of its atoms or groups of atoms, and in the process is broken down into positively and negatively charged particles.

Electron, an elementary unit of electricity; negatively charged particle of the atom.

Electron Microscope, an optical instrument using a beam of electrons directed through an object to produce an enlarged image (up to $100,000 \times$ magnification) on a fluorescent screen or photographic plate.

Electroshock, shock produced by electric current.

Electrotherapy, treatment of disease by use of electricity.

Electuary, soft, medicated confection.

Elephantiasis, tropical disease in which blocking of the lymph vessels by a parasite leads to great swelling of the tissues, especially in the lower part of the body.

Elimination, discharge of indigestible materials and waste products from the body.

Elixer, a sweetened, alcoholic liquid used to disguise unpleasant tasting medicines.

Emaciated, excessively thin.

Emasculation, castration.

Embalming, preservation of a corpse against decomposition.

Embolism, small clot or foreign substance detached from the inside of a blood vessel and floating free in the blood stream.

Embolus, a blood clot (or other substance such as air, fat, or tumor) inside a blood vessel, where it becomes an obstruction to circulation.

Embryo, earliest stage of development of a young organism; the human young through the third month of pregnancy.

Embryology, the study of the development of embryos.

Emedullate, to deprive of marrow.

Emesis, vomiting.

Emetic, drug that causes vomiting.

Emetine, drug that causes sweating and expectoration.

Emiction, urination.

Emission, sending forth; discharge of semen.

Emmenia, the menses.

Emmenology, that which is known about mestruation.

Emmenagogue, that which stimulates the menstrual flow.

Emollient, relaxing, soothing agent used to soften the skin or internally to soothe an irritated surface.

Emotion, mental attitude.

Empathy, understanding, sympathy.

Emphysema, lung disease characterized by the thinning and loss of elasticity of lung tissue.

Emphiric, based on experience.

Empyema, collection of pus in the lung.

Emulgent, draining out.

Emulsion, product made up of tiny globules of one liquid suspended in another liquid.

Enamel, the hard, white substance which covers and protects the tooth.

Encelialgia, pain in abdominal region.

Encephalic, pertaining to the brain.

Encephalitis, inflammation of the brain.

Encephalogram, brain x-ray.

Encephalomalacia, softening of the brain due to deficient blood supply.

Encephalon, the brain.

Encranial, located within the cranium.

Endangium, membrane which lines blood vessels.

Endeictic, symptomatic.

Endemic, a term used to describe a disease that is constantly present in or native to a particular region or locality.

Endermic, administered through the skin.

Endoblast, cell nucleus.

Endocardial, pertaining to the interior of the heart.

Endocarditis, inflammation of the inner lining of the heart, especially the heart valves.

Endocardium, tissue lining the inside of the heart.

Endochrome, coloring matter of a cell.

Endocranial, within the cranium.

Endocrine Glands, ductless glands that secrete directly into the blood stream.

Endocrinology, study of ductless glands and their secretions.

Endoderm, inner layer of cells of an embryo.

Endodontitis, inflammation of the dental pulp.

Endometritis, inflammation of the lining of the womb.

Endometrium, tissue that lines the interior wall of the womb.

Endomoeba, a single-celled parasite that lives in humans.

Endoplast, nucleus of a cell.

End-Organ, any terminal structure of a nerve.

Endothelium, the thin lining of the blood vessels.

End Pleasure, pleasure enjoyed at the height of the sexual act.

End Product, the final excretory product that passes from the system.

Endothermic, characterized by heat absorption.

Enema, an injection of liquid into the rectum, usually intended for the treatment of constipation.

Energy, ability to work.

Enervation, weakness.

Engorgement, excessive fulness.

Engram, the indelible impression which experience makes upon nerve cells.

Enomania, craving for alcoholic drink, delerium tremens.

Enstrophe, turning inward.

Ental, inner.

Entamoeba, a microscopic ameba.

Enteralgia, pain in the intestine.

Enteric, pertaining to the intestines.

Enteritis, inflammation of the intestinal tract by infection or irritating food.

Enterocolitus, inflammation of the small and large intestines.

Enteron, the intestine.

Enthetic, introduced from without.

Entopic, located in the proper place.

Entropian, turning in of the edge of the eyelid so that the lashes rub against the eyeball.

Enucleate, to remove a tumor or an organ in its entirety.

Enuresis, bed wetting.

Environment, external surroundings.

Enzyme, a substance produced by living cells which, although not participating in a chemical reaction, promotes its speed.

Ephebic, pertaining to puberty.

Ephedrine, drug used to shrink the lining of the nose in colds and in the treatment of asthma.

Ephelis, freckle.

Ephidrosis, profuse sweating.

Epibular, upon the eyeball.

Epicutaneous, on the surface of the skin.

Epicyte, wall of a cell.

Epicardium, the outer layer of the heart wall. It is also called the visceral pericardium.

Epidemic, disease that affects many people at one time in the same area.

Epidemic Pleurodynia, an epidemic disease caused by a virus. The disease causes pain in the region of the chest or abdomen, as well as fever. One of the typical symptoms of epidemic pleurodynia is a relapse occurring two to three days after the original attack. Epidemic pleurodynia is also referred to as Bornholm's disease.

Epidemiology, study of the occurrence and distribution of disease.

Epidermis, outermost layer of the skin.

Epididymitis, inflammation of the epididymis, a structure which covers the upper end of the testicle.

Epiglottis, a lid which covers the opening to the windpipe and prevents food from getting into the voice box or lungs.

Epilation, removal of hair by the root.

Epilepsy, a symptom of some disorder in the brain. The name of this condition comes from the Greek word for seizure. The brain has many millions of nerve cells, called neurons, that work together to control or guide the actions of the body. To do their work; the nerve cells build up a supply of electricity through the action of the chemicals they contain. Each cell has its own storage battery, which it discharges at the proper moment and then recharges instantaneously.
However, cells can become overactive and fire off irregularly. This distrubance can suddenly spread to neighboring areas or jump to distant ones or even overwhelm the brain. When it spreads, a seizure results. The great majority of the neurons soon begin working in harmony again, and the seizure is over.
Epilepsy is a condition in which seizures occur. A seizure itself is the sign of an abnormal release of energy within the brain.
There are three major types of epilepsy: grand mal, petit mal, and focal seizures.

Epinephrine, the active principle of one of the secretions of the adrenal gland.

Epiotic, located on or above the ear.

Epiphora, continuous overflow of tears.

Episiotomy, cutting of the wall of the vagina during childbirth to avoid tearing.

Epistasis, substance which rises to the surface instead of sinking.

Epistaxis, nose bleeding.

Epithelioma, cancer of the skin.

Epithelium, cellular substance of skin and mucous membrane.

Eponym, using the name of a person to designate a disease, organ, syndrome, etc.

Equilibrium, balance.

Equivalent, of equal value.

Erasion, abrasion.

Erection, becoming upright and rigid.

Eremophobia, extreme fear of being alone.

Erepsin, intestinal enzyme.

Erg, unit of work.

Ergasiatrics, psychiatry.

Ergophobia, extreme fear of work.

Ergosterole, substance found in the skin and elsewhere which, when exposed to sunlight, becomes converted to vitamin D.

Ergot, drug used to cause contraction of the uterus and control bleeding after childbirth.

Ergotamine, an alkaloid substance used in treatment of migraine and can produce contractions of the uterus.

Erode, wear away.

Erogenous, producing sexual excitement.

Erosion, wearing away of a substance.

Erotic, pertaining to sex.

Erotogenic, originating from sexual desire.

Erotogenic Zones, areas of the body, stimulation of which promote sexual feelings.

Erotophobia, extreme fear of sexual love.

Errhine, causing sneezing and nasal discharge.

Eructation, belching.

Eruption, rash; cutting of a tooth.

Erysipelas, infection of the skin with streptococci.

Erythema, redness of the skin.

Erythema Multiforme, one of the more severe forms of oral ulcerations. Because the skin and the mucous lining of the mouth are similar in structure, the same kind of sores will develop both on the skin and in the mouth. Erythema multiforme is common in children and young adults. It appears most frequently in the winter and spring months.

Erythroblastosis, a condition brought about by an incompatibility of Rh factors. The condition can cause severe anemia and a failing heart.

Erythrocytes, red blood cells.

Erythroderma, skin disturbance characterized by abnormal redness.

Erythromycin, an antibiotic drug with many of the same properties as penicillin.

Esbach's Method, a method of estimating quantity of albumin in urine.

Eschar, sloughed tissue due to a burn.

Esophagus, the tube that connects the stomach to the throat, about nine inches long.

Essential Hypertension, an elevated blood pressure not caused by kidney or other evident disease. Sometimes called primary hypertension, it is commonly known as high blood pressure.

Ester, compound formed by the combination of an organic acid with an alcohol.

Estrogens, female sex hormones. Estrogens have special importance at puberty, because they are responsible for the development of secondary sex characteristics—such as the growth of the breast. Estrogens also stimulate the growth of the lining of the uterus. Any hormone that affects the monthly cycle of changes taking place in the female genital tract is considered to be an estrogen.

Estrus, female sexual cycle.

Estuarium, vapor bath.

Ether, organic liquid used as an anesthetic.

Ethics, Medical, system of moral principles governing medical conduct.

Ethnic, pertaining to the races of mankind.

Etiology, study of the causes of disease.

Eucalyptus, an oil used as an antiseptic in nasal solutions and mouth washes.

Eugenics, study of inheritance.

Eunuch, castrated male.

Eupepsia, normal digestion.

Euphonia, normal clear condition of the voice.

Euphoria, exaggerated sense of well-being.

Eupnea, normal respiration.

Eusitia, normal appetite.

Eustachian Tube, the tube that connects the pharynx with the middle ear.

Euthanasia, mercy killing.

Evacuant, medicine which empties an organ; laxative.

Evagination, protusion of a part or organ.

Eversion, turning outward.

Evisceration, removal of inner parts.

Evolution, gradual transition from one state to another.

Ex- (prefix), out; away from.

Exacerbation, increase in the degree of sickness.

Examination, scrutiny of a patient's state of health.

Exanthema, any fever accompanied by a rash.

Excerebration, removal of the brain.

Excise, surgical removal.

Excitability, susceptible to stimulation.

Excitation, stimulation; irritation.

Excoriation, rubbing away of part of the skin by disease or injury.

Excrement, feces.

Excretory Systems, the several different systems that eliminate waste products that enter or are formed within the body.

Exenteration, evisceration.

Exercise, physical exertion.

Exhalation, expulsion of air from the lungs.

Exhaustion, extreme fatigue.

Exhibitionist, abnormal impulse to show one's genitals to a member of the opposite sex.

Exhilarant, cheering.

Exo- (prefix), outside; outward.

Exocardia, abnormal position of the heart.

Exocrine Glands, glands that have ducts and that deliver their secretions to a specific location.

Exodontia, tooth extraction.

Exophthalmos, bulging of the eyes, usually caused by over-activity of the thyroid gland.

Exostosis, outgrowth from the surface of a bone.

Expansion, increase in size.

Expectorant, drug supposed to have the effect of liquefying the sputum.

Expectoration, spittle.

Expire, exhale; die.

Exploration, investigation.

Expression, the act of squeezing out; facial disclosure of feeling or emotion.

Exterior, outside.

Extern, medical student who works in a hospital but lives elsewhere.

Extima, outermost covering of a blood vessel.

Extirpation, complete surgical removal or destruction of a part.

Extra- (prefix), outside of; in addition.

Extracorporeal Circulation, the circulation of the blood outside the body as by a mechanical pump-oxygenator.

Extract, to pull out; remove the active portion of a drug.

Extrasystole, a contraction of the heart that occurs prematurely and interrupts the normal rhythm.

Extremity, terminal part of anything; a limb of the body.

Extrinsic, of external origin.

Extrovert, one interested in external objects and actions.

Eye, the organ of vision. The eye is a hollow ball or globe that contains various structures that perform specific functions. The bulb of the eye, or eyeball, is composed of three layers of tissue.

Eyebrow, hair ridge above the eye.

Eyeground, the inside of the back part of the eye seen by looking through the pupil.

Eyelash, hair growing on the edge of an eyelid.

Eyestrain, eye fatigue.

Eyetooth, a cuspid or upper canine tooth.

— F —

F., Fahrenheit, one gauge of measuring temperature.

Face, anterior part of the head.

Facial, pertaining to the face.

Facies, appearance of the face.

Facilitation, hastening of a natural process.

Facioplegia, facial paralysis.

Factitious, artificial.

Faculty, normal power or function; mental attribute.

Fahrenheit Scale, boiling point of water 212 degrees, freezing point, 32 degrees.

Fahr., Fahrenheit.

Fainting, temporary loss of consciousness due to insufficient blood reaching the brain. Fainting is a mild form of physical shock. It may be caused by an injury, the sight of blood, exhaustion, weakness, lack of air, and emotional shocks such as fright.
The patient feels weak and becomes dizzy, black spots appear before his eyes, his face becomes pale and his lips blue, and his forehead is covered with perspiration. He then sinks back in his seat or falls to the ground unconscious. The pulse is rapid and weak, and the breathing is shallow. The above symptoms usually occur in a few seconds.

Fallopian Tubes, tubes which connect the ovaries with the womb.

Fallout, settling of radioactive dust from the atmosphere after a nuclear explosion.

False, not true.

False Labor, early contractions over a period of several hours or even days during pregnancy.

False Ribs, lower five pairs of ribs.

Familial, pertaining to the same family.

Family, group descended from a common ancestor.

Fang, root of a tooth.

Farina, meal; flour.

Far Point, farthest point which an eye can see distinctly when completely relaxed.

Farsightedness, difficulty in close vision.

Fastigium, acme; highest point.

Fat, obese; greasy deposits in body tissue.

69

Fatigue, exhaustion; weariness.

Fauces, space in the back part of the mouth, surrounded by the soft palate, the tonsil arches and the base of the tongue.

Favus, contagious skin disease.

F.D., fatal disease.

Fear, emotional response to danger.

Fear Reaction, emotional illness in which anxiety is shown by the conscious fear of a particular event or object.

Febricide, that which destroys fever.

Febrifacient, producing fever.

Febrile, pertaining to fever.

Febris, fever.

Fecal, pertaining to feces.

Feces, waste matter excreted by the bowels.

Fecundity, fertility.

Feeble-mindedness, state of low development of the intelligence.

Feeding, taking of food.

Fee Splitting, unethical practice of dividing the patient's charges between the referring physician and the consultant.

Feet, the extremities of the legs on which humans stand.

Fellatio, type of sexual perversion in which the male sex organ is placed in the mouth of another.

Felon, deep skin, infection on the far end and inner surface of a finger.

Female, woman; girl; pertaining to a woman.

Feminism, possession of female characteristics by a male.

Femoral Artery, the main blood vessel supplying blood to the leg.

Femur, thighbone. It is the longest and strongest bone in the body. The femur extends from the hip joint to the knee. Its upper end is rounded to fit into the socket in the pelvis, and the lower end broadens out to help form the knee joint.

Fenestration, surgical operation designed for the treatment of certain types of deafness.

Fermentation, decomposition of complex substances under the influence of enzymes.

Ferrule, metal band applied to a tooth to strengthen it.

Fertile, capable of reproduction.

Fertilization, the union of a spermatozoa (male sex cell) and an ovum (female sex cell).

Fester, to produce pus.

Fetal, pertaining to a fetus.

Fetation, pregnancy.

Feticide, killing of an unborn child.

Fetid, having a disagreeable odor.

Fetish, that which becomes attractive because of its association with sexual pleasure.

Fetus, an unborn child from the third month until birth.

Fever, elevation of the body temperature.

Fiber, threadlike structure.

Fibrillation, state of tremor in the muscles found in certain nervous, muscular and heart diseases. When filbrillation occurs, it is often necessary to use a defibrillator, such as electric shock, to stop the uncoordinated contractions and restore the normal heartbeat.

Fibrin, protein substance produced by elements of the blood and tissues which forms a network as the base of clots.

Fibrinogen, a soluble protein in the blood which, by the action of certain enzymes, is converted into the insoluble protein of a blood clot.

Fibrinolysin, an enzyme that can cause coagulated blood to return to a liquid state.

Fibroid, benign tumor of the womb consisting of tough, fibrous tissue.

Fibroidectomy, surgical removal of a fibroid tumor.

Fibroma, benign tumor composed of fibrous tissue.

Fibrositis, the commonest rheumatic condition that does not affect the joints directly.

Fibrous Tissue, two types of connective tissue, both composed of fibrous cells. White fibrous tissue is dense and helps form tendons and ligaments. Yellow fibrous tissue is not as dense as white fibrous tissue. It is more elastic and can be found in arterial walls.

Fibula, bone of lower leg.

Filament, small, threadlike structure.

Field, limited area.

Figure, body; shape; outline.

Filament, delicate fiber or thread.

Filariasis, tropical disease due to infection of the body with tiny worms which block the lymph vessels, causing swelling of the limbs, elephantiasis.

Filling, material inserted in the cavity of a tooth.

Filter, to pass a liquid through a porous substance to eliminate solid particles; device used in this process.

Filtrate, fluid which has passed through a filter.

Finger, digit of the hand.

First Aid, emergency, temporary medical care and treatment of an injured person. The aim of first aid is to prevent death or further injury, to relieve pain, and to counteract shock until medical aid can be obtained.

Fission, division into parts.

Fissure, groove, cleft.

Fistula, abnormal passage leading from the surface of the body to an internal cavity.

Fit, convulsion; sudden attack.

Flaccid, flabby; weak; soft.

Flagellation, to beat or whip; beating as a means of satisfying sexual desires.

Flap, mass of partly detached tissue.

Flat Foot, not having the normal arch of the sole of the foot.

Flatulence, gas in the stomach or intestines. This causes a very uncomfortable feeling. Although flatulence can be caused by diseases and by fermentation in the intestines, it is usually the result of swallowing air. The patient feels that he can relieve the discomfort by burping, but actually all he does is swallow more air. This is a very typical cycle seen in nervous patients.

Flatus, stomach or intestinal gas.

Flaxseed, linseed.

Fleas, small, wingless insects that feed on the blood of animals and humans.

Flesh, soft tissue and muscles of the animal body.

Fletcherism, thorough mastication of food.

Flex, to bend.

Flexion, bending.

Flexor, muscle that bends or flexes.

Floating, moving around; out of normal position.

Flora, plant life.

Florid, having a bright color.

Fl. Oz., fluid ounce.

Fluid, a non-solid, liquid or gaseous substance.

Fluorescent Antibody Test, a rapid and sensitive test for certain disease organisms and substances. Its value in the field of heart disease is that it speeds the recognition of harmful streptococci in a throat smear, so that immediate treatment might avert an attack of rheumatic fever. The test consists of "tagging" with a fluorescent dye the antibodies, i.e., substances in blood serum that have been built up against certain bacteria. This dyed antibody is then mixed with a smear taken from the throat of the patient. If streptococci are present in the smear, the glowing antibodies will attach to them, and they can be clearly seen in the microscope.

Fluoride, a mineral that is important for sound tooth development and for the prevention of tooth decay.

Fluoroscope, an X-ray instrument used to examine the interior of the body.

Fluoroscopy, the examination of a structure deep in the body by means of observing the fluorescence on a screen, caused by X-rays transmitted through the body.

Flush, to blush; to clean with a stream of water.

Flutter, irregular, rapid motion; agitation, especially of the heart.

Flux, a large flow of any body excretion, particularly the bowel contents.

Fly, the housefly. This fly is a danger to the health of man and animals, principally because it carries and spreads disease germs that may be in the materials it breeds in, feeds on, or walks on.

Focal Seizures, some types of epilepsy in which abnormal electrical discharges can be traced to one small area, or focus, in the brain, or to a number of such areas.

Fold, ridge; a doubling back.

Folie, mania; psychosis.

Follicle, small secretory sac or gland.

Folliculitis, inflammation of the follicles of the hair.

Fomentation, treatment of inflammation by applying heat and moisture to the affected part.

Fontanel, the soft spot of a baby's head that later is closed by the growth of bone.

Food, that which nourishes—the body's source of energy. Food is necessary to support growth, to repair constantly wearing tissues, and to supply energy for physical activity. Unless the food consumed supplies all the elements required for normal life processes, the human body cannot operate at peak efficiency for very long. If an essential nutrient is missing from the diet over very long periods of time, "deficiency diseases" such as rickets, scurvy, or certain anemias may develop.

Food Allergies, allergies caused by sensitivity to one or more foods. The symptoms, which can appear shortly after the food is eaten, affect the skin, the digestive tract, or the respiratory system.

Food Poisoning, digestive disorder due to eating foods containing poisonous substances.

Foot, terminal part of the leg.

Foot Print, impression of the foot.

Foramen, any opening or perforation.

Foramen Ovale, an oval hole between the left and right upper chambers of the heart that normally closes shortly after birth.

Forceps, two-pronged instrument for extracting.

Forearm, portion of the arm between the elbow and wrist.

Forefinger, first finger.

Forehead, portion of the head above the eyes; brow.

Forensic Medicine, aspects of medicine related to law.

Formation, structure; shape; figure.

Formula, rule prescribing the kind and quantity of ingredients in a preparation.

Fornication, sexual intercourse of persons not married to each other.

Fossa, pit; depression.

Fracture, a break in a bone. There are two main kinds of fractures. A simple fracture is one in which the injury is entirely internal—that is, the bone is broken but there is no break in the skin. In simple fractures there is no considerable displacement of the ends of the broken bone.

A compound fracture is one in which there is an open wound in the soft tissues and the skin. Sometimes the open wound is made when a sharp end of the broken bone pushes out through the tissues and skin; sometimes it is made by an object piercing the skin and tissues and breaking the bone.

Compound fractures are more serious than simple fractures. They usually involve extensive damage to the tissues, and they are quite likely to become infected.

Fragilitas, brittleness.

Fragility, characteristic of being easily broken.

Frenum, fold of skin or lining tissue that limits the movement of an organ, e.g., tissue under the tongue.

Freckles, small patches of pigmented skin more commonly found in blonde or red-headed people.

Freezing, frigidity of a limb due to severe cold.

Frenzy, maniacal excitement.

Friable, easily broken into small pieces.

Friction, rubbing.

Friedman's test, a test for pregnancy that involves injecting the woman's urine into a rabbit.

Fright, extreme, sudden fear.

Frigidity, absence of sexual desire in women, coldness.

Frons, forehead.

Frontal, relating to the front of the body or an organ; pertaining to the forehead.

Frost Bite, condition caused by long exposure to severe cold; freezing of a part of the body, usually nose, fingers, toes. At first the symptoms are burning, stinging, and then numbness. However, the victim may not be aware of frostbite of the cheeks, ears, or nose until someone tells him, or of frostbite of hands or feet until he removes his gloves or shoes.

Ice crystals in the skin cause a gray or white waxy color, but the skin will move over bony ridges. When the part is completely frozen, there are ice crystals in the entire thickness of the extremity, indicated by a pale, yellow, waxy color. The skin will not move over bony ridges. When the frozen part is thawed, it becomes red and swollen, and large blisters develop.

Frottage, rubbing, massage.

Fructose, a simple sugar that resembles glucose.

Frustration, the feeling aroused when physical or personal desires are thwarted.

Fugitive, wandering.

Fulguration, therapeutic destruction of tissue by means of electric sparks.

Fulling, kneading.

Full Term, normal end of pregnancy.

Fumes, vapors.

Fumigation, disinfecting.

Function, normal and specific action of a part.

Fundament, base; foundation.

Fundus, base of an organ.

Fundus of the Eye, the inside of the back part of the eye, seen by looking through the pupil. Examining the fundus of the eye is used as a means of assessing changes in the blood vessels. The fundus of the eye is also called the eyeground.

Fungicide, an agent that destroys fungi.

Fungus, mold.

Funny Bone, outer part of the elbow which is crossed by part of the ulnar nerve.

Fur, deposit forming on the tongue.

Furfur, dandruff.

Furibund, maniacal.

Furor, rage.

Furuncle, boil.

Furunculosis, boils on skin.

Fusiform, spindle-shaped.

Fusion, uniting.

Gait, manner of walking.

Galactic, pertaining to milk.

Galactischia, suppression of the secretion of milk.

Galactorrhea, excessive flow of milk.

Galactosemia, an inherited disorder caused by a missing enzyme necessary for the digestion of milk or lactose to convert galactose into the useful glucose of the blood.

Galeophobia, extreme fear of cats.

Gall, secretion stored in the liver which helps in emulsifying fats.

Gall Bladder, sac beneath the liver which stores bile and secretes mucus.

Gallop Rhythm, an extra, clearly heard heart sound that, when the heart rate is fast, resembles a horse's gallop.

Gall Stones, stone-like objects found in gall bladder and its drainage system, composed primarily of calcium.
If a large stone starts to move, its possessor will know that something is radically wrong. The movement of the stone may cause an attack of severe pain. One may suddenly feel a stabbing pain in the upper right portion of the abdomen. The pain may spread out—it may be felt on both sides, in the back, throughout the abdomen, where it shifts from side to side, and it may be felt in the right shoulder. This pain is often so intense that the sufferer may be in agony. He becomes wet with perspiration; he may vomit. Often he has a chill with a high fever. The upper right quarter of his abdomen may become very tender to pressure. An attack of this kind may be over in a few minutes or it may last a week.
If a gallstone is so located as to cause obstruction to the flow of bile into the intestine, the person may become yellow (jaundiced). An individual may have only one attack, or he may have several attacks at irregular intervals.

Galvanism, uninterrupted electric current.

Gamete, a female or male reproductive or sex cell; i.e., an ovum or a sperm.

Gammacism, imperfect pronunciation of g and k sounds.

Gamma Globulin, a type of protein in the blood that aids the body in resisting diseases.

Gamogenesis, sexual reproduction.

Gamophobia, extreme fear of marriage.

Ganglion, cyst-like swelling found in the region of a joint or the sheath of a tendon; area between two nerve fibers.

Ganglionic Blocking Agent, a drug that blocks the transmission of a nerve impulse at the nerve centers (ganglia).

Gangrene, death and deterioration of a part of the body, caused by interference with the blood supply.

Gapes, disease of fowls caused by a worm.

Gargle, mouth wash.

Gargoylism, a form of dwarfism with heavy facial features, damaged vision, and mental retardation.

Gastralgia, stomach pain.

Gastrectomy, the surgical removal of all or a portion of the stomach.

Gastric, pertaining to the stomach.

Gastritis, inflammation of the stomach walls.

Gastrobrosis, perforation of the stomach.

Gastrocnemius, calf muscle.

Gastroenteritis, inflammation of the stomach and intestine.

Gastroptosis, abnormal relaxation of stomach musculature.

Gastrorrhagia, stomach hemorrhage.

Gastrosis, any stomach disease.

Gatophilia, abnormal fondness for cats.

Gatophobia, extreme fear of cats.

Gaucher's Disease, a family disease, particularly found in Jewish families. The onset of Gaucher's disease occurs in infancy and consists of listlessness, bronze spots in the skin, retardation, and eventual paralysis. No specific treatment is yet available. The disease is also known as familial splenic anemia.

Gauntlet, hand bandage.

Gavagi, liquid nourishment supplied through a tube inserted into the mouth, down the gullet and into the stomach.

Gelatin, body protein in a solid state, used in manufacture of drug capsules.

Gelatinous, like jelly.

Gelosis, hard, swollen mass.

Gelotolepsy, spontaneous loss of normal muscle tension.

Geminate, in pairs.

Gen., gene.

Genal, pertaining to the cheek.

Gender, sexual category; male or female.

Gene, biological unit which transmits hereditary characteristics.

Generation, reproduction; period of family history.

Generative, pertaining to reproduction.

Generic, pertaining to genus; distinctive.

Genesis, origin and development.

Genetics, the science of natural differences and similarities in successive generations of living organisms.

Genetous, dating from fetal life.

Genial, pertaining to the chin.

Genicular, pertaining to the knee.

Genital, pertaining to the sex organs.

Genitalia, reproductive organs.

Genitourinary System, the genital and urinary system.

Genocide, race destruction.

Genu, knee; knee-like structure.

Genus, biological classification.

Geophagy, eating of soil.

Geriatic, pertaining to old age.

Geriatrics, medical study of old age.

Germ, organism that infects man; primitive beginning of a developing embryo.

German Measles, a viral infection characterized by high fever and skin rash. German measles is also known as rubella.

Germicide, agent that destroys germs.

Geroderma, wrinkling of the skin.

Gestation, pregnancy.

Gestosis, toxemia in pregnancy.

Gibbous, humpbacked.

Gigantism, abnormal height and size.

Gingiva, the gum that surrounds the tooth.

Gingivitis, inflammation of the gums.

Girdle, encircling structure.

Glabella, space between the eyebrows.

Glabrous, smooth.

Gladiolus, main portion of the sternum.

Glanders, contagious horse disease.

Glandilemma, outer covering of a gland.

Glandula, small gland.

Glands, there are three main types of glands: the lymph glands, which are found mainly at various junctions in the body, such as the armpit and the groin, and also within the body and around the base of the neck, their function being to trap germs and prevent them from reaching vital areas; larger glands, such as the pancreas and liver which produce digestive agents such as bile, enzymes, etc. and which empty their products into the intestines through a duct or tube; the endocrine glands, which are also called ductless glands because they empty their products directly into the blood stream.

Glandular, pertaining to a gland.

Glandule, small gland.

Glans, cone-shaped body that forms the tip of the penis or clitoris.

Glasses, lenses to aid vision.

Glaucoma, disease of the eyes in which the pressure of the fluid in the eye increases. Prolonged high eye pressure can kill many nerve fibers in the eyes. Once destroyed, these nerve fibers are never usuable again. The increased eye pressure, called increased intraocular pressure, strangles the optic (eye) nerve and the blood vessels that nourish it. A block in normal eye drainage is the usual cause of such increased pressure.

Gleet, discharge from the urethra found in chronic gonorrhea.

Glioma, tumor of the nerve cells.

Globular, spherical.

Globule, small droplet.

Globulicidal, destroying red corpuscles.

Globulin, the name of a group of proteins.

Globus, ball, sphere.

Globus Hystericus, imaginary lump in the throat.

Glomerulonephritis, kidney disease.

Glomerulus, small, round mass; important element of the kidney.

Glossa, tongue.

Glossalgia, tongue pain.

Glossitis, inflammation of the tongue.

Glottis, the space between the vocal cords.

Glucohemia, sugar in the blood.

Glucose, liquid which is sweet and important to body chemistry; sugar.

Gluteal, pertaining to the buttocks.

Gluten, protein, found in cereals.

Glutinous, sticky.

Glycemia, sugar in the blood.

Glycerin, clear, syrupy liquid used for medicinal purposes.

Glycolysis, digestion of sugar.

Glycosuria, sugar in the urine.

Glycyrrhyza, licorice.

Gnathic, pertaining to the jaw.

Gnosia, faculty of perception and recognition.

Goiter, an enlargement of the thyroid gland. It is usually caused by lack of iodine in the diet, but in some areas of the world goiter also may be caused by certain agents in the food. The number of cases in the United States and in many other countries has been greatly reduced in recent years by adding iodine to table salt.

Goitrogenic, causing goiter.

Gold, a heavy metal that is used as a drug to treat certain diseases and conditions.

Gomphiasis, looseness of teeth.

Gonad, ovary or testes.

Gonadotrophin, hormone which stimulates the ovary or testes.

Gonagra, gout in the knee.

Gonalgia, pain in the knee.

Gonococcus, germ which causes gonorrhea.

Gonorrhea, veneral disease.

Gouge, instrument for cutting bone.

Gout, disease in which there is an upset in the metabolism of uric acid, causing symptoms of joint pain.

Gouty, pertaining to gout.

G.P., general practitioner.

Gracile, slender.

Gradatim, gradually.

Graft, piece of tissue for transplantation. The areas most frequently used to remove skin for a graft are the legs and the back of the neck.
The grafted area takes the place of the scar that would normally form. The advantage of the skin graft (aside from the cosmetic value) is that a grafted area will be more flexible than a scarred area.

Grand Mal, epileptic attack.

Granulation, process of wound healing.

Granulocytopenia, disease which reduces the defensive cells in the blood, the white blood cells.

Granum, grain.

Grave's Disease, increased activity of thyroid gland with bulging of the eyes.

Gravid, pregnant.

Gravida, pregnant woman.

Gravity, weight.

Gray Matter, a slang term used to indicate the brain. The term is applicable because most of the brain belongs to the nervous system, and most nerve tissues are gray in color.

Grip, influenza; grasp.

Groin, depression between the thigh and abdomen.

Grumous, lumpy; clotted.

G.U., genitourinary.

Gumboil, a swelling in the mouth due to an abscess at the root of a tooth.

Guilt, feeling of having committed an offense.

Gullet, passage to the stomach.

Gums, the tissues and membrane surrounding the teeth.

Gun-Barrel Vision, vision in which the field is narrow, as if the patient were looking through a tube. The visual field is the total area perceived when the eyes are focused straight ahead. This comprises both the small area on which the eyes are focused for sharp impression (central vision) and the large area that is seen "out of the corner of the eye" (indirect or peripheral vision).

In gun-barrel vision, the eye loses the ability to see "out of the corner of the eye"; that is, the eye loses the peripheral vision. Gun-barrel vision is also called shaft vision or tunnel vision.

Gustation, sense of taste.

Gustatory, pertaining to the sense of taste.

Gut, bowel; intestine.

Gutta, a drop.

Guttate, like a drop.

Guttur, throat.

Guttural, pertaining to the throat.

Gymnastics, physical exercise.

Gymnophobia, extreme fear of the naked body.

Gymandromorphism, condition in which one has male and female characteristics.

Gynatrisia, condition in which there is no passageway in the vagina.

Gynecic, pertaining to women.

Gynecoid, like a woman.

Gynecologist, specialist in female diseases.

Gynecology, study of the diseases of women.

Gynecomastia, enlargement of male breasts.

Gynoplasty, plastic surgery of the female genitals.

Gyrus, one of the convolutions of the cerebral cortex of the brain.

— H —

Habit, automatic action; bodily temperament.

Habituation, becoming accustomed to a thing.

Hachement, hacking.

Hacking, chopping stroke in massage.

Hair, threadlike outgrowth from the skin.

Halazone, white powder used as drinking water disinfectant.

Halitosis, offensive breath.

Halitous, covered with moisture.

Hallucination, mistaken sense impression.

Hallucinogens, drugs capable of provoking changes of sensation, thinking, self-awareness and emotion.

Hallucinosis, condition of persistent hallucinations.

Hallux, big toe.

Ham, back part of the thigh above the knee and below the buttock; hip, thigh; buttock.

Hamarthritis, arthritis in all the joints.

Hammer, instrument for striking blows; middle ear bone.

Hammer Toe, claw-like deformity of the toe.

Hamster, rodent frequently used in laboratory tests.

Hamstring Muscles, the collection of muscles at the back of either thigh.

Hamular, hook-shaped.

Hand, terminal part of an arm.

Handedness, tendency to use a particular hand.

Hangnail, partly detached piece of skin at the root of a fingernail.

Hangover, the body's reaction to an excess of alcohol. The associated symptoms of nausea, gastritis, anxiety, and headache vary by individual.

Haphiphobia, extreme fear of contact.

Haptics, science of the sense of touch.

Hare Lip, cleft lip.

Haunch, hips and buttocks.

Haut-Mal, epileptic attack at its peak.

Hay Fever, an allergic disease caused by abnormal sensitivity to certain air borne pollens.

84

HB., hemoglobin.

Head, a nonmedical term used to indicate the part of the body above the neck, including the face, brain, ears, etc.

Headache, a pain that lasts several minutes or hours; it may cover the whole head, one side of it, or sometimes the front or the back of the head. The pain may be steady or throbbing, barely noticeable, or completely prostrating. To add to the confusion about a definition, some people call any dizzy, tense, or queer feeling in the head a headache. Doctors feel that headache is not a disease by itself but rather a symptom. Headache is important because it can be the symptom—perhaps the first warning—of a serious condition that probably could be controlled if detected early. Headache may be classified as acute or chronic. The acute headache occurs suddenly and occasionally and is an unpleasant part of many illnesses. Chronic headaches recur more or less frequently.

Heal, cure.

Healing, process of making well.

Health, state of having a normally active body and mind.

Hearing, perceiving sound.

Hearing Aid, device used by one who is deaf to amplify sound waves.

Hearing Impairments, hearing losses. There are two main types of hearing loss—conductive deafness and perceptive or nerve deafness. Conductive deafness exists when sound waves are blocked before they reach the inner ear. Perceptive or nerve deafness, which is much more serious, results when there is a defect in the inner ear or when there is damage to the nerve that carries the impulses to the brain, or injury to the brain itself.

Heart, the powerful, muscular, contractile organ, the center of the circulatory system.

By its pump action, the heart keeps the blood under pressure and in constant circulation throughout the body. In a healthy person, with the body at rest, the heart contracts about seventy-two times a minute. This varies with age, weight, sex, amount of exercise, and body temperature. Each contraction of the heart is followed by limited relaxation. Cardiac muscle never completely relaxes but always maintains a degree of tone. Contraction of the heart is systole and is the period of work. Relaxation of the heart with limited dilation is called diastole and is the period of rest. A complete cardiac cycle is the time from the onset of one contraction or heartbeat to the onset of the next.

Heart Attack, a serious decrease in the flow of blood to the heart muscle.

Heart Block, disease of the heart in which the impulse of contraction is unable to pass from the auricles to the ventricles, with the result that both beat independently of each other.

Heartburn, burning sensation, either in the back of the throat or in the left side of the chest, usually occurs after eating.

Heart Failure, inability of the heart to maintain adequate body ciculation.

Heart-Lung Machine, a machine through which the bloodstream is diverted for pumping and oxygenation while the heart is opened for surgery.

Heart Murmur, abnormal heart sound.

Heart Rate, number of heart beats per minute.

Heart Transplant, an operation that replaces a severely diseased or malfunctioning heart with a healthy heart.

Heat, warmth; high temperature; form of energy; sexual excitement in certain animals; to make hot.

Heat Cramps, painful spasms of muscles, especially those of the abdomen and limbs, after prolonged exposure to high temperatures while engaged in strenuous labor.

Heat Exhaustion, collapse from the effects of heat from the sun or any other source. It occurs more frequently when the humidity is high.
The patient is seldom unconscious but may complain of feeling very weak. His face is pale and anxious-looking and covered with cold perspiration. Frequently he vomits. He may complain of feeling chilly. His pulse is rapid and weak, and his breathing is shallow, with little chest expansion.

Heatstroke, state of dizziness, nausea and spots before the eyes due to direct exposure to high temperatures.

Hebetic, pertaining to puberty.

Hebetude, mental slowness.

Hectic, habitual; constitutional.

Hedonism, devotion to pleasure.

Heel, hind extremity of the foot.

Heimlich Maneuver, method for helping a choking victim. The method involves grasping the victim from behind with the fist against the victim's abdomen and the other hand holding the fist and pressing upward into the abdominal area with a sharp movement.

Helcoid, resembling an ulcer.

Helcosis, formation of an ulcer.

Helicine, spiral.

Heliosis, sunstroke.

Heliotherapy, treatment of disease by the rays of the sun or by the use of an ultra violet-lamp.

Heliotropism, tendency of an organism to turn toward sunlight.

Helix, margin of the external ear.

Helminthiasis, presence of parasitic worms in the body.

Heloma, callosity, corn.

Helotomy, surgical removal of a corn.

Hemafacient, blood producing agent.

Hemagogue, agent which promotes the flow of blood.

Hemangiectasis, enlargement of blood vessels.

Hemarthrosis, accumulation of blood in a joint.

Hemase, blood enzyme.

Hematemesis, vomiting of blood.

Hematic, pertaining to blood.

Hematischesis, stopping of bleeding.

Hematocolpos, collection of blood in the vagina.

Hematoid, resembling blood.

Hematologist, one who specializes in the study of blood and its diseases.

Hematology, science of the blood.

Hematoma, swelling containing clotted blood, usually caused by direct violence, e.g., a black eye.

Hematometachysis, blood transfusion.

Hematonosis, blood disease.

Hematuria, the passing of blood in the urine.

Hemeralopia, day blindness.

Hemi-(prefix), half.

Hemianopsia, blindness in half of the visual field of each eye.

Hemic, pertaining to blood.

Hemicrania, headache on one side of the head only; migraine.

Hemifacial, affecting one side of the face.

Hemiplegia, paralysis of one side of the body caused by damage to the opposite side of the brain. The paralyzed arm and leg are opposite to the side of the brain damage because the nerves cross in the brain, and one side of the brain controls the opposite side of the body. Such paralysis is sometimes caused by a blood clot or hemorrhage in a blood vessel in the brain.

Hemocidal, destructive of blood cells.

Hemocyte, blood corpuscle.

Hemodynamics, the study of the flow of blood and the forces involved.

Hemofuscin, brown coloring matter of blood.

Hemoglobin, the oxygen-carrying red-colored substance of the red blood cells. Hemoglobin carries oxygen to the body tissues. If the amount of hemoglobin is below normal, not enough oxygen will get to the tissues. When hemoglobin has absorbed oxygen in the lungs, it is bright red and is called oxyhemoglobin. After it has released the oxygen load in the tissues, it is purple in color and is called reduced hemoglobin.

Hemoid, resembling blood.

Hemolysis, destruction of elements of the blood.

Hemopathy, blood disease.

Hemopericardium, blood in the heart sac

Hemopexin, blood coagulating enzyme.

Hemopexis, coagulation of blood.

Hemophilia, blood disease characterized by defective coagulation of the blood and a strong tendency to bleed.
Hemophilia, or bleeder's disease, is the commonest of a rather rare, incurable group of hereditary blood disorders occurring almost exclusively in males but transmitted through women. Females themselves generally show no signs of difficulty.

Hemophiliac, one afflicted with hemophilia.

Hemophobia, aversion to blood.

Hemophoris, conveying blood.

Hemoptysis, spitting up of blood.

Hemorrhage, severe loss of blood from a blood vessel. In external hemorrhage, blood escapes from the body. In internal hemorrhage, blood passes into tissues surrounding the ruptured blood vessel. Hemorrhage (escape of blood) occurs whenever there is a break in the wall of one or more blood vessels. In most small cuts, only capillaries are injured. Deeper wounds result in injury to veins or arteries. Bleeding that is severe enough to endanger life seldom occurs except when arteries or veins are cut.

Hemorrhagenic, causing hemorrhage.

Hemorrhoids, enlarged, dilated veins inside or just outside the rectum. Hemorrhoids are also called piles. They are somewhat like varicose veins in the legs. The veins in the rectum are not buried deep in the flesh but lie close to the surface, where they can easily be pressed on and irritated. Any pressure that slows up the flow of blood through them or that irritates can cause piles.

Hemopasia, withdrawal of blood.

Hemostasis, stopping of hemmorhage.

Hemostat, instrument which stops bleeding, clamp.

Hemotherapy, using blood to treat disease.

Hemothorax, accumulation of blood between the lungs and chest wall.

Hepar, liver.

Heparin, substance which prevents clotting of blood.

Hepatic, concerning the liver.

Hepatitis, a swelling and soreness of the liver. Two types caused by viruses—infectious and serum hepatitis—are frequently found in the United States. One is called "infectious" because a person with the disease can infect others by contact. This type is also spread by contaminated water and food, including raw clams and oysters harvested from polluted waters. "Serum" hepatitis was first recognized in people who had been given medicines or vaccines that contained human serum. A person may develop serum hepatitis after receiving a transfusion of infected blood or its derivatives or after having contaminated needles, syringes, or other skin-puncturing instruments (including tattoo needles) used on him.

Hepatogenic, produced in the liver.

Hepatoma, tumor with its origin in the liver.

Hepatomegaly, enlargement of the liver.

Hepatopathy, liver disease.

Hereditary, transmitted from one's forefathers.

Heredity, traits and characteristics transmitted from parents and other ancestors to offspring.

Heredosyphilis, congenital syphilis.

Hermaphodite, one having both male and female sex characteristics.

Hermetic, Hermetical, airtight.

Hernia, rupture; the bulging out of a part of any of the internal organs through a weak area in the muscular wall.

Heroin, morphine chemically altered to make it three to six times stronger. Heroin is an addictive narcotic (a drug that relieves pain and induces sleep).

Herpes, skin disease characterized by clusters of small blisters.

Herpes Simplex, fever blisters, mouth blisters.

Herpes Simplex Type II (genital herpes), a viral infection transmitted through sexual intercourse.

Herpes Zoster, acute, infectious, inflammatory skin disease; shingles.

Herpetiform, resembling herpes.

Heterogeneous, of unlike natures.

Heterosexuality, sexual desire for one of the opposite sex.

Hexamethonium Chloride, a drug that lowers blood pressure and increases blood flow by interfering with the transmission of nerve impulses that constrict the blood vessels.

Hiatus, fissure, gap.

Hiccups, sharp, inspiratory sound caused by contractions of the diaphragm.
Hiccups can often be stopped by increasing the amount of carbon dioxide in the system. This can be accomplished by rapidly drinking a glass of water or by breathing into a paper bag. When the underlying cause is more serious, stronger measures may have to be taken.

Hidrosis, sweating.

Hip, upper part of the thigh where it joins with the pelvis.

Hippocrates, Greek physician, the Father of Medicine.

Hippocratic Oath, oath taken by the graduating physician on which he bases his medical ethics.

Hirsute, hairy.

Histamine, bodily substance found in most tissues, released when tissue is damaged.

Histoblast, tissue cell.

Histology, science of the microscopic structure of tissues.

Histoma, any tissue tumor.

History, patient's record of past illness, present illness and symptoms.

Hitch, knot.

HIV (human immunodeficiency virus), virus which causes AIDS.

Hives, skin rash characterized by large wheals.

Hoarseness, difficulty in speaking.

Hodgkin's Disease, disease in which the lymph glands and spleen become enlarged.

Holarthritis, inflammation of all joints.

Homeopathy, a method of treating diseases that involves giving the patient a minute dose of a drug that normally causes symptoms similar to his own.

Homogeneous, of uniform structure.

Homosexuality, psychological disorder which causes one to be attracted to people of same sex.

Hook, curved instrument used for traction or holding.

Hookworm Disease, a disease caused by microscopic worms. The most common way of getting hookworm disease is by walking barefoot on infected soil or by handling such dirt. Once the hookworms are in the body, they are carried by the blood to the heart and then to the lungs. There they bore through the membranes and get into the bronchial tubes and are coughed up into the throat. Even if some are expectorated, others are swallowed. Those that are swallowed go down through the stomach to the intestines, where they stay.
Hookworm disease makes a person listless and weak, even in mild cases.

Hordeolum, sty.

Hormone, a chemical that originates in the glands and is carried to all parts of the body by the blood.

Horror, fear, dread.

Hospital, institution for the care of those in need of medical attention.

Hospitalization, placing of a person in a hospital for treatment.

Host, organism on which a parasite lives.

Hot, having a high temperature.

Hot Flashes, sudden attacks of feeling hot, flushing, and sweating, characteristic of menopause.

Hottentotism, abnormal form of stuttering.

House Physician, doctor who lives in the hospital and is available for help at all times.

House Staff, residents, interns and certain doctors of a hospital.

Humerus, arm bone.

Humidifier, device used to increase moisture in the air of a room.

Humidity, amount of moisture in the air.

Humor, body fluid.

Humpback, curvature of the spine.

Hunger, desire, especially for food.

Huntington's Chorea, a rather rare inherited disease.

Hyaline, glassy.

Hybrid, product of parents of different species.

Hydatid, cyst formed in the tissues.

Hydragogue, strong laxative.

Hydralazine Hydrochloride, a drug that lowers blood pressure. An antihypertensive agent.

Hydrarthrosis, accumulation of fluid in a joint.

Hydroa, skin disease with blisterlike patches.

Hydrocarbon, compound of hydrogen and carbon.

Hydrocephalus, abnormal enlargement of the head due to interference with the drainage of cerebral fluid.

Hydrocyst, cyst with watery contents.

Hydrogenate, combine with water.

Hydrogen Peroxide, a strong antiseptic.

Hydrophilia, absorbing water.

Hydrophobia, rabies.

Hydrops, dropsy.

Hydrotherapy, treatment of disease by means of water.

Hygiene, science of health and observance of its rules.

Hygienic, pertaining to health.

Hygiene, Mental, development and preservation of mental health.

Hygiene, Oral, proper care of the mouth and teeth.

Hygienist, specialist in hygiene.

Hymen, membrane fold located at the entrance to the female sex organs.

Hymenectomy, surgical removal of the hymen.

Hymenotomy, surgical opening of the hymen.

Hypacusia, faulty hearing.

Hypalgesia, reduced sensitivity to pain.

Hyper, a prefix meaning too much or too high.

Hyperacidity, excess of stomach acid.

Hyperacuity, sharp vision.

Hyperacusia, acute hearing.

Hyperbulia, excessive willfulness.

Hypercholesteremia, an excess of a fatty substance called cholesterol in the blood.

Hyperemesis, abnormal amount of vomiting.

Hyperglycemia, excess blood sugar.

Hyperhydrosis, excessive sweating.

Hypermastia, unusually large breasts; having more than two breasts.

Hypermotility, increased activity.

Hyperopia, farsightedness. A condition in which far vision is very good but near or close vision is poor because the focus of light rays is behind the retina.

Hyperplasia, an abnormal increase of the number of normal cells. Hyperplasia is frequently the result of a hormone imbalance.

Hyperpresia, unusually high blood pressure.

Hyperpnea, hard breathing with an increase in the depth of inhalation.

Hyperrhinolalia, marked nasal quality of the voice.

Hypersensitivity, allergy.

Hypersthenia, unusual strength or tone of body.

Hypertension, high blood pressure.
Primary hypertension, the most common kind of high blood pressure, apparently is not related to any other disease and its cause is not known. Secondary hypertension is high blood pressure caused by an underlying disease.
Treatment which varies with causes and individual cases, may include surgery, drugs, weight reduction or other dietary restriction, or a combination of these.

Hyperthermia, abnormally high temperature.

Hyperthymia, excessive emotionalism.

Hyperthyroidism, condition caused by excessive secretion of the thyroid gland.

Hypertrichosis, excessive hairiness.

Hypertrophy, the enlargement of a tissue or organ owing to an increase in the size of its constituent cells.

Hypnagogic, causing sleep.

Hypnagia, pain while asleep.

Hypnogenetic, causing sleep.

Hypnosis, trance induced through verbal suggestion or concentration upon an object.

Hypnotherapy, treatment by hypnotism.

Hypnotic, any drug that induces sleep.

Hypnotize, to put in a state of hypnosis.

Hypo, a prefix meaning too little or too low.

Hypobaropathy, decompression sickness.

Hypocalcia, calcium deficiency.

Hypochondria, undue concern about one's health; suffering with imaginary illnesses.

Hypochondriac, one who suffers from imaginary illness.

Hypodermic, beneath the skin; injection under the skin; needle used for injections.

Hypogastrium, lowest middle abdominal region.

Hypoglobulia, decrease of red blood cells.

Hypoglossal, under the tongue.

Hypoglycemia, a condition in which the level of blood sugar is abnormally low or abnormally reduced. Hypoglycemia may be caused by many different factors.

Hypogonadism, deficient activity of testis or ovary.

Hypomastia, unusual smallness of the breast.

Hypomenorrhea, deficient menstruation.

Hyponoia, mental sluggishness.

Hypophrenia, feeblemindedness.

Hypopraxia, deficient activity.

Hypophysis, pituitary gland.

Hypoplasia, incomplete tissue development.

Hyposensitization, treatment of allergy by giving small doses of the material to which the person is allergic and gradually increasing the doses until the allergic reaction is reduced.

Hypotension, low blood pressure.

Hypothalamus, the part of the brain that exerts control over activity of the abdominal organs, water balance, temperature, etc.

Hypothesis, supposition.

Hypothyroidism, a condition in which the thyroid gland is underactive, resulting in the slowing down of many of the body processes, including the heart rate.

Hypotonia, abnormally low strength or tension.

Hypoxia, a condition in which there is less than the normal content of oxygen in the organs and tissues of the body.

Hysterectomy, surgical removal of whole or part of the womb.

Hysteria, psychological state or neurosis resulting from failure to face reality.

Hysterosalpingectomy, surgical removal of the womb and fallopian tubes.

Iateria, therapeutics.

Iatric, medical.

Iatrogenic, a term that literally means "caused by the doctor." A patient's belief that he has a disease or condition that is based solely on the physician's actions, manner, or other clues belongs in this category. An iatrogenic illness is based on the power of suggestion. The term is also used to indicate any condition that follows or results from the treatment given a patient by a physician.

Iatrogenic Disease, condition caused by a doctor's statements or procedure.

Iatrology, medical science.

Ice, frozen water.

Ichnogram, footprint.

Ichor, watery discharge from a sore.

Ichthyol, coal tar product used in the treatment of skin diseases.

Iconologny, sexual desire aroused by pictures or statues.

Icthyophobia, extreme fear of fish.

Ichthyosis, condition in which babies have dry and scaly skin.

Icterpatitis, jaundice.

Icteric, relating to or characterized by jaundice.

Icterus, jaundice.

Ictus, beat; stroke; attack.

Id, psychological term for the unconscious.

Idea, concept.

Idea, Flight of, rapid, disconnected speech characteristic of certain mental diseases.

Ideal, concept of perfection.

Ideation, thinking.

Idée Fixe, obsession.

Identical, exactly the same.

Identical Twins, twins developed from one fertilized cell.

Idiosyncrasy, peculiar characteristics whereby one person differs from another.

Idiocrasy, peculiarity.

Idiocy, mental deficiency with an I.Q. under 25.

Idiogamist, man capable of having sexual relations only with his wife, or only with a few women.

Idiot, person suffering from congenital feeblemindedness.

Idiotic, like an idiot.

Idiotypic, relating to heredity.

Idrosis, excessive sweating.

Ignis, cautery.

Ileitis, inflammation of the lower small intestine.

Ileocolitis, inflammation of the lower small intestine and the large intestine.

Ileum, lower part of the small intestine.

Ileus, intestinal obstruction.

Iliac Artery, a large artery that conducts blood to the pelvis and the legs.

Ilium, flank, upper wide part of the hipbone.

Ill, not healthy; diseased.

Illegal, not lawful.

Illegitimate, not according to law; born out of wedlock.

Illness, ailment.

Illusion, misinterpretation of a real sensation.

Imagery, imagination.

Imago, memory of a loved person formed in childhood.

Imbalance, lack of balance.

Imbecility, mental deficiency with the mental age between three and seven years and an I.Q. between 25 and 49.

Imbibation, absorption of a liquid.

Imbrication, surgical procedure for closing wounds.

Immature, not fully developed.

Immedicable, incurable.

Immersion, placing a body under a liquid.

Immersion Foot, a condition caused by exposure to cold water (50°F. and below) for twelve hours or more or to water of approximately 70°F. for several days. Inability to move about freely is also a contributing factor. These injuries are characterized by tingling and numbness, swelling of the legs and feet, bluish discoloration of the skin, and by blisters and pain.
The best treatment is to expose the affected areas to warm, dry air.

Immiscible, not able to be mixed.

Immobilization, making immovable.

Immune, protected against disease.

Immunity, ability to resist infectious disease. When an individual's own body provides immunity automatically, he is said to have a natural immunity to a specific disease.
There are two types of active acquired immunity. In one type, the person produces the antibodies (defensive agents) to defend the body. This often occurs after a person has had a particular disease—such as measles. In this type of immunity, one attack of the disease confers immunity against subsequent attacks. Another type of active acquired immunity is artificially induced. This is done by injecting the individual with weakened or dead bacteria or viruses. This method is known as vaccination or immunization. The amount of bacteria or viruses is enough to force the body to develop antibodies against the injected substance but not strong enough to actually give the individual the disease. In this way the body is prepared to defend itself against the stronger form of the same disease.
Passive acquired immunity is obtained by injecting foreign antibodies into an individual. These antibodies usually come from an animal that has been vaccinated. This form of immunity is important in cases where an individual has already been exposed to a disease and needs immediate protection. Passive acquired immunity may be used against diseases such as tetanus and diphtheria.

Immunization, the process of artificially conferring immunity to a specific disease.

Immunologist, one who specializes in the science of immunity.

Immunology, science dealing with the study of the processes by which the body fights infection.

Impacted Teeth, teeth that cannot grow properly because of the angle at which they are growing.

Impaction, firmly wedged in.

Impalpable, too weak or fine to be felt.

Impar, unequal.

Imperative, obligatory, involuntary.

Impermeable, not allowing to pass through.

Impervious, unable to be penetrated.

Impetigo, infectious disease of the skin characterized by isolated pustules.
Impetigo spreads easily from one person to another and from one part of the body to other parts. The open sores contain germs that transfer the infection.

Implant, graft, insert.

Implantation, the attachment of the fertilized egg into the lining of the uterus.

Impotence, sexual weakness in the male.

Impotent, unable to copulate; sterile.

Impregnation, fertilization; saturation.

Impulse, instinctual urge.

Inanimate, lifeless.

Inanition, starvation.

Inarticulate, without joints; not given to clear expression.

Inborn, innate; inherent.

Inbreeding, mating between close relatives.

Incest, sexual relations between those of close relationship.

Incidence, the number of new cases of a disease developing in a given population during a specific period of time, such as a year.

Incipient, beginning; about to appear.

Incision, a wound made by a sharp cutting instrument such as a knife, razor, broken glass, etc. Incisions, commonly called cuts, tend to bleed freely, because the blood vessels are cut straight across. There is relatively little damage to the surrounding tissues. Of all classes of wounds, incisions are least likely to become infected, because the free flow of blood washes out many of the microorganisms (germs) that cause infection.
The term incision is also used to indicate a surgical stroke that cuts open part of the body.

Incisor, any one of the four front teeth of either jaw.

Inclination, tendency.

Incompetent, not functioning properly.

Incompetent Valve, any valve that does not close completely and consequently allows blood to leak or flow back in the wrong direction.

Incontinency, inability to control evacuation.

Increment, increase.

Incretion, internal secretion.

Incrustation, scab.

Incubate, to provide favorable conditions for growth and development.

Incubation, stage of an infectious disease from the time the germ enters the body until the appearance of the first symptoms. During the early incubation period of a contagious disease the patient is not usually contagious; however, toward the end of the incubation period he may be highly contagious.
The incubation period of a disease varies considerably. Bacterial diseases such as diphtheria usually have shorter incubation periods than do diseases, such as chickenpox, that are caused by viruses. The two major exceptions to this are the common cold and influenza.

Incubator, a piece of equipment that is used to protect premature babies.

Incubus, nightmare.

Incurable, not able to be cured.

Index, forefinger.

Indication, any aspect of a disease that points out its treatment.

Indigenous, native to a particular place.

Indigestion, failure of digestive function; a somewhat vague term used to indicate a wide variety of uncomfortable stomach symptoms. Flatulence, nausea, heartburn, and other similar symptoms are often classified as indigestion.
Indigestion may be a symptom of a serious disorder, or it may simply be caused by overeating. Indigestion frequently results from eating when emotionally upset or when rushed. At these times much of the blood leaves the digestive tract, as a result of strong emotion or for use by the muscles. Without a sufficient supply of blood, the digestive organs cannot perform properly. The result may be indigestion.

Indolent, inactive.

Induced, brought about by indirect stimulation.

Indurated, hardened.

Inebriation, intoxication.

Inert, inactive.

Inertia, inactivity.

In Extremis, at the point of death.

Infant, baby.

Infanticide, killing of an infant.

Infantile, pertaining to infancy; possessing characteristics of early childhood.

Infantile Paralysis, infection of central nervous system; poliomyelitis.

Infantilism, failure of development.

Infarct, an area of tissue that is damaged or dies as a result of not receiving a sufficient blood supply. The term is frequently used in the phrase "myocardial infarct," referring to an area of the heart muscle damaged or killed by an insufficient flow of blood through the coronary arteries that normally supply it.

Infarction, blockage of a vessel.

Infection, the invasion of the body by harmful microorganisms. Any break in the skin or other body membrane (such as the mucous membrane that lines the nasal passages) is dangerous, because it allows microorganisms (germs) to enter the wound. Although infection may occur in any wound, it is a particular danger in wounds that do not bleed freely, wounds in which torn tissue or skin falls back into place and so prevents the entrance of air, and wounds that involve crushing of the tissues. Incisions, in which there is a free flow of blood and relatively little crushing of the tissues, are least likely to become infected. Infections are dangerous in any part of the body but particularly so in the area around the nose and mouth. From this area infections spread very easily into the bloodstream, causing septicemia (blood poisoning), and into the brain, causing abscesses and infections there. Boils, carbuncles, and infected hair follicles just inside the nostril are perhaps the most common infections that occur in this area. The general symptoms of infection include heat, redness, swelling, and pain around the wound or site of the infection. Pus is often (although not always) visible. If the infection is severe, there may be an increase of body temperature and swelling of the glands in the neck, armpit, or groin. Infections are usually treated with antibiotics.

Infectious, liable to be transmitted by infection.

Infectious Mononucleosis, an infectious disease. The major characteristic of infectious mononucleosis is constant fatigue. In addition, possible symptoms include fever (although this may be only a low, persistent fever), headache, sore throat, swollen glands, jaundice, and upset stomach.

One of the major problems with mononucleosis is the difficulty involved in proper diagnosis. Because the symptoms are fairly general, special tests must be made to diagnose infectious mononucleosis. The problem is further complicated because not all patients have the symptoms.

The incubation period for infectious mononucleosis is between five and fifteen days. Patients are contagious for two to four weeks, but, since the method of transmission is not clear, the amount of time a patient is contagious is sometimes difficult to gauge.

Inferior, of a lower position or situation.

Infertility, sterility.

Infiltration, process by which substances pass into cells or into the spaces around cells.

Infirm, weak, feeble.

Infirmary, place for the care of the sick.

Infirmity, weakness, sickness.

Inflammation, changes that occur in living tissues when they are invaded by germs, e.g. redness, swelling, pain and heat.

When a part of the body is attacked by foreign organisms, the injured cells in the area release a substance called histamine. The histamine forces the blood vessels in the area to expand, thus increasing the flow of blood and fluid. This increase causes the redness, heat, and swelling. The additional fluid and swelling increase the pressure in the area and cause the pain associated with inflammation.

Inflation, distention.

Inflection, bending inward.

Influenza, virus infection characterized by fever, inflammation of the nose, larynx and bronchi, neuralgic and muscular pains and gastrointestinal disorder.

There are several known main types of influenza virus. Each type has various strains, and each is somewhat different from the others. Sometimes new strains develop. These are very likely to cause epidemics, because people have had no experiences with them to help build up some degree of natural immunity against them. Because existing vaccines are ineffective against new virus strains, a special vaccine has to be developed, usually on short notice, to protect the susceptible population. Single cases of influenza appear occasionally, but the disease usually occurs in epidemic form.

Influenza attacks suddenly. The symptoms can be some or all of the following: fever, chills, headache, sore throat, cough, and soreness and aches in the back and limbs. Although the fever usually lasts only one to five days, the patient is often as exhausted or weakened as if he had gone through a long illness. No known medicine will cure influenza.

Infracostal, below a rib.

Infracture, incomplete bone fracture.

Inframaxillary, below the jaw.

Infrared, beyond the red portion of the visible spectrum.

Ingestion, taking by mouth; eating; drinking.

Ingravescent, gradually becoming worse.

Inguinal, referring to the groin.

Inhalant, that which is inhaled.

Inhalation, taking of air into the lungs.

Inherent, intrinsic, innate.

Inherited, received from one's ancestors.

Inhibition, restraint.

Initial, beginning; first; commencing.

Initis, inflammation of muscular substance.

Injection, forcing a liquid into body tissue or a cavity.

Injury, hurt; damage.

Inlay, filling for a dental cavity.

Inlet, means of entrance.

Innate, hereditary; congenital.

Innervation, distribution of nerves to a part; amount of nervous stimulation received by a part.

Innocent, harmless; benign.

Innocuous, harmless.

Innominate, nameless.

Innominate Artery, one of the largest branches of the aorta. It rises from the arch of the aorta and divides to form the right common carotid artery and the right subclavian artery.

Inoculation, immunization against disease by introducing one form of the germ or its products into the body.

Inoculum, material used in inoculation.

Inoperable, not surgically curable.

Inorganic, without organs; not of organic origin.

Inquest, medical examination of a corpse to determine cause of death.

Insanity, mental disorder.

Insatiable, not able to be satisfied.

Inscription, part of a prescription which states the names and amounts of ingredients.

Insect Bites and Stings, the injection of a toxic substance into the body by an insect. Many insects bite or sting, but few are poisonous in the sense that their bite or sting can cause serious symptoms of itself. However, there are insects that do transmit diseases; these insects act as hosts to an organism or virus of diseases. For example, certain types of mosquitoes transmit malaria, yellow fever, and other diseases; certain types of ticks transmit spotted or Rocky Mountain fever; and certain types of biting flies transmit tularemia or rabbit fever. Occasionally, stinging or biting insects have been feeding on or in contact with poisonous substances, and at the time of the sting or bite such substances may be injected into or come in contact with the wound thus made, causing a poisoned or infected wound.

Insecticide, agent which kills insects.

Insemination, fertilization of the female by introduction of male sperm.

Insensible, not perceived by the senses; unconscious.

Insheathed, enclosed.

Insidious, stealthy; applied to a disease that does not show early symptoms of its advent.

Insipid, without taste; without animation.

In Situ, in the normal place.

Insoluble, not capable of being dissolved.

Insomnia, the inability to sleep. Insomnia may be caused by external sources such as noise, an unfamiliar bed, excessive heat or cold, etc. Pain can also cause insomnia. Surprisingly, being too tired (either mentally or physically) can also interfere with getting to sleep. Overstimulation from coffee and tea keep some people awake. One of the most common causes of insomnia is emotional upset. Physicians try to cure the cause of insomnia rather than try to cure the insomnia itself.

Inspection, visual examination.

Inspersion, sprinkle with powder or fluid.

Inspiration, breathing in.

Inspissated, thickened.

Instillation, pouring a liquid by drops.

Instinct, inherent behaviour pattern.

Insufficiency, incompetency. In the term valvular insufficiency, it means an improper closing of the valves, which admits a backflow of blood in the wrong direction. In the term myocardial insufficiency, it means the inability of the heart muscle to do a normal pumping job.

Insulin, internal secretion of the pancreas concerned with metabolism of glucose in the body. When there is a lack of insulin or the body is not using insulin properly, unused sugar collects in the blood. This condition is called diabetes.

Integration, assimilation.

Integument, skin.

Intellect, mind.

Intelligence, ability to see the relationship between things.

Interatrial Septum, the muscular wall that divides the left and right upper chambers of the heart, which are called atria.

Intercellular, between the cells.

Intercostal, between two ribs.

Intercourse, communication between persons.

Intercourse, Sexual, coitus.

Intermittent Claudication, pain in legs after brief exercise caused by a defect in blood circulation.

Intern, an assistant physician of a hospital staff who is in training prior to receiving a license to practice medicine.

Internist, doctor who specializes in diseases of the internal organs.

Internship, term of service of an intern.

Internus, internal.

Interstice, space or gap in a tissue or structure.

Intertrigo, an acute skin irritation and inflammation.

Intervascular, between blood vessels.

Interventricular Septum, the muscular wall, thinner at the top, that divides the left and right lower chambers of the heart, which are called ventricles.

Intestinal, pertaining to the intestines.

Intestine, the digestive tract beginning at the mouth and ending at the anus.

The intestines are composed of two major parts: the small intestines and the large intestines. The names "small" and "large" refer to the diameter of the tubes. In a living body, the small intestine is only five or six feet long. However, after death, the contraction relaxes, and it becomes apparent that the small intestine is actually about twenty-two feet long. In contrast, the large intestine is only five feet long. The intestines finish the digestive process begun in the stomach and prepare the waste products for excretion from the body.

Intima, innermost covering of a blood vessel.

Intolerance, not able to endure.

Intoxication, drunkenness.

Intra-Abdominal, within the abdomen.

Intracapsular, within a capsule.

Intrad, inwardly.

Intramuscular; within the muscular substance.

Intravenous, within a vein.

Intravital, during life.

Intrinsic, innate.

Introvert, one whose thoughts and interests are turned inward upon himself.

Intuition, instinctual knowledge.

Intussusception, a condition in which a segment of the intestine will fold in on itself, cutting off the passageway.

Inunction, massaging the skin with an ointment.

Invagination, becoming insheathed.

Invalid, one who is sickly.

Inversion, turning inside out.

Inversion, Sexual, homosexuality.

Invertebrate, having no backbone.

Invest, enclose.

Inveterate, hard to cure.

In Vitro, process or reaction that is carried out in laboratory test tube; a term used to indicate a phenomenon studied outside a living body under laboratory conditions. In vitro literally means "in glass," hence in a laboratory vessel.

In Vivo, within the living organism.

Involution, return to normal that certain organs undergo after fulfilling their function, e.g., the breast after breast feeding; period of decline after middle age.

Iodine, chemical element used as an antiseptic and therapeutic agent in medicine; a naturally occurring mineral that is necessary for the proper functioning of the thyroid gland. People who live away from the seacoast in areas where the soil is low in iodine sometimes fail to get an adequate supply of this mineral. Getting too little iodine can cause, goiter, a swelling of the thyroid gland.
Iodized salt and seafoods are reliable sources of iodine. Regular use of iodized salt is the most practical way to assure enough iodine in the diet.

Ionizing Radiation, radiation that tears molecules apart, leaving their fragments electrically charged.

Iophobia, extreme fear of poisons.

Ipecac, died plant root used against dysentery and as an emetic; expectorant and diaphoretic.

Ipsilateral, situated on the same side.

I.Q., intelligence quotient.

Iridial, pertaining to the iris.

Iridectomy, surgical removal of the iris, the colored portion of the eye.

Iris, colored portion of the eye.

Iritis, inflammation of the iris.

Iron, chemical element found mainly in the hemoglobin of the red blood cell; a metallic element that is needed by the body in relatively small but vital amounts. Iron combines with protein to make hemoglobin, the red substance of blood that carries oxygen from the lungs to body cells and removes carbon dioxide from the cells. Iron also helps the cells obtain energy from food. Because of the normal monthly blood loss (menstruation), women need twice the amount of iron that men do. Only a few foods contain much iron. Liver is a particularly good source. Lean meats, heart, kidney, shellfish, dry beans, dry peas, dark-green vegetables, dried fruit, egg yolk, and molasses also count as good sources. Whole-grain and enriched bread and cereals contain smaller amounts of iron, but when eaten frequently they become important sources.

Iron Lung, respirator; apparatus to aid breathing.

Irritable, capable of reacting to a stimulus; sensitive to stimuli.

Irritants, substances that do not directly destroy the body tissues but cause inflammation in the area of contact.

Ischemia, a local, usually temporary, deficiency of blood in some part of the body. Ischemia is often caused by a constriction or an obstruction in the blood vessel suplying that part of the body.

Ischium, bone upon which body rests when sitting.

Ischuria, retention of urine.

Islets of Langerhans, groups of specialized cells scattered throughout the pancreas. These special cells produce insulin.

-ism, (suffix), condition; theory; method.

Isocellular, composed of identical cells.

Isolation, separation of persons having a contagious disease.

Isotope, a term applied to one of two elements, chemically identical, but differing in some other characteristic, such as radioactivity.

Issue, offspring; suppurating sore kept open by a foreign body in the tissue.

Isthmus, neck or narrow part of an organ.

Itching, annoying skin sensation relieved by scratching.

Iter, tubular passage.

-itis (suffix), inflammation.

IUD (intrauterine device), method of birth control which requires the insertion of a small piece of molded plastic or copper into the uterus.

I.V., intravenously.

Ixodic, pertaining to or caused by ticks.

Jacket, covering for the thorax; plaster of Paris or leather bandage used to immobilize spine or correct deformities.

Jacksonian Seizure, a type of focal seizure caused by some types of epilepsy. It is the result of overactive nerve cells in the part of the brain that controls the movement of muscles. The seizure usually begins in the fingers or toes of one hand or foot, or sometimes in the corner of the mouth. The affected part trembles violently or perhaps becomes numb. As more nerve cells become affected, the trembling or numbness spreads. It may stop as suddenly as it began, or it may spread to the other side of the body. When the seizure spreads, the patient loses consciousness and has an attack similar to grand mal (another type of epilepsy).

Jactitation, convulsive movements; restless tossing.

Jail Fever, typhus fever.

Jargon, incoherent speech.

Jaundice, increase in bile pigment in blood causing yellow tinge to skin, membranes and eyes; can be caused by disease of liver, gallbladder, bile system or blood.

Jaw, applied to one of two bones that form the skeleton of the mouth.

Jecur, the liver.

Jejunitis, inflammation of the jejunum.

Jejunum, middle section of the small intestine.

Jelly, thick, homogeneous mass.

Jerk, abrupt muscular movement.

Jockey Strap, suspensory, scrotum support.

Joint, the place where two or more bones or cartilage come together. There are several types of joints, but there are two major classifications: immovable joints, such as the bones in the head; and movable joints, such as the elbow.
Movable joints are protected against friction by cartilage and by special fluids. The fluid is contained in small pockets or bursae. If the cartilage or bursae are injured or diseased, movement in the joint is limited and very painful. There are four types of movable joints in the human body.
The ball-and-socket joint includes a rounded end of bone that fits into a pocket, or socket, of another bone. The joints between the thighbone and the hip and be-

tween the upper arm and the shoulder are ball-and-socket joints. A hinge joint unites two bones in an arrangement similar to a door hinge, allowing movement chiefly within an up-and-down or back-and-forth area. Examples of hinge joints are the elbow and the knee. A pivotal joint, such as in the lower arm, is one in which one bone rolls or rotates over another bone. A gliding joint permits two bones to slide or glide over each other. The ankle and wrist are two examples of gliding joints.

Jugal, pertaining to the cheek or bone.

Jugular Vein, large vein at front of throat.

Juice, body secretions.

Junction, point of meeting or coming together.

June Cold, rose fever.

Jungle Rot, tropical fungus infection.

Justo Major, larger than normal.

Justo Minor, smaller than normal.

Juvenile, pertaining to youth; young; immature.

Juxtaposition, placed side by side; close together.

Juxtaspinal, near the spinal column.

Kaif, tranquid state caused by drugs.

Kainophobia, extreme fear of new things.

Kakosmia, foul odor.

Kakotrophy, malnutrition.

Kala-Azar, disease which occurs in tropical countries and shows itself in fever, anemia, dropsy and swelling of the liver and spleen.

Kali, potash.

Kanamycin, a broad-spectrum antibiotic.

Kaolin, powdered aluminum silicate used for ulcerations, wounds that discharge freely or internally for inflammation of the intestines.

Karezza, prolonged sexual intercourse without ejaculation.

Karyogenesis, formation and development of a cell nucleus.

Karyomorphism, the form of a cell nucleus.

Karyon, cell nucleus.

Kata- (prefix), down.

Katabolism, breaking down process in metabolism.

Keloid, large scar formation.

Kelosteroid, group of chemical substances produced by the body of primary importance to normal development, body functioning and life.

Kelotomy, relief of hernia strangulation by incision.

Kenophobia, extreme fear of empty spaces.

Kephalin, commercial remedy for headache.

Kephyr, type of fermented milk.

Keratalgia, pain in the cornea.

Keratectomy, surgical removal of part of the cornea.

Keratin, the protein that is the principal component of nails, hair, and epidermis.

Keratitis, inflammation of the cornea.

Keratoiritis, inflammation of both the cornea and iris.

Keratolytic, agent that causes skin to shed.

Keratoma, horny growth.

Keratosis, any skin disease that causes an overgrowth of a horny material, e.g., multiple warts.

Kernicterus, a condition of severe mental retardation that results from a blood incompatability involving the Rh blood factor.

Sometimes the blood of a pregnant woman will start to build up immunity against any conflicting blood type of her unborn child. A couple who have a potential blood conflict can have from one to five normal children before the increasing blood-sensitivity of the mother threatens to cause kernicterus in her child.

This disorder used to be responsible for an estimated one percent of the severely retarded in institutions; yet it can usually be prevented by treatment. Through repeated blood transfusions for the baby before or at birth, the exchange transfusions can wash out the hostile sensitized blood before brain damage occurs.

Rh-negative mothers may become sensitized to Rh-positive blood from having an Rh-positive baby, an Rh-positive miscarriage, or an accidental Rh-positive blood transfusion.

Kidney, two small but vital organs of the human body. A little larger than a man's fist and roughly bean-shaped, the kidneys lie in the small of the back on each side of the spine. They remove waste products from the blood and regulate the amount of water and the delicate balance of chemical substances in the body. These intricate functions are absolutely essential to human life. The kidneys also assist in regulating the production of red blood cells, which carry vital oxygen from the lungs to all parts of the body, and in maintaining normal blood pressure. The life of every human being depends as much on his kidneys as on his lungs or his heart. About nineteen gallons of blood pass through the kidneys every hour. On the average, a person's entire blood supply is filtered through the kidneys twenty to twenty-five times per day. Within the outermost layers (the cortex) of the kidney the blood passes through an intricate network of arteries. These arteries grow progressively smaller, ending in microscopic units called nephrons. A single kidney contains almost a million nephrons, each of them part of a filtering system that removes fluid containing waste products brought from all parts of the body by the blood. This is the first step in the complex function of the kidneys.

This waste-carrying fluid, called filtrate, is still rich in minerals and protein. Passing from the nephrons into an arrangement of coiled tubes, most of the filtrate and its essential minerals and proteins are absorbed back into the blood. This process takes place in the medulla. The liquid remaining after these two steps have been completed is called urine. Urine collects in a pouch called the pelvis in the center of the kidney. From each kidney a tube called a ureter carries the urine to the bladder, where it is stored until it is discharged through another tube, the urethra. The entire system is called the urinary tract.

Kilo, one thousand.

Kilogram, one thousand grams.

Kilnemia, blood output of the heart.

Kinematics, science of motion.

Kinesia, motion sickness.

Kinesis, motion.

Kinesthesia, the muscle sense.

Kinesthetic Sensations, the electrical impulses sent to the central nervous system by the nerves in muscles.

Kinetic, pertaining to motion.

Kink, bend; twist.

Kleptomania, obsessive stealing.

Kleptophobia, fear of stealing.

Knee, the point of juncture of the femur and tibia.

Kneecap, patella.

Knock Knee, condition when legs are turned in at knees.

Knot, knoblike structure; small nodule.

Kolp- (prefix), vagina.

Kolpitis, inflammation of the vagina.

Kopiopia, eyestrain.

Kraurosis, dryness and hardening of skin.

Kreotoxism, meat poisoning.

Kresol, germicide.

Kwashiorkor, a syndrome or set of widely recognized symptoms caused by malnutrition, specifically a lack of protein and amino acids.

Kyllosis, clubfoot.

Kymoscope, apparatus for measuring blood pressure variations.

Kyogenic, causing pregnancy.

Kyphosis, a condition in which the vertebral column (the spine) is abnormally curved in the chest area.

Labial, pertaining to a lip.

Labialism, speech defect with the use of labial sounds.

Labile, changeable; unsteady.

Lability, instability.

Labiology, study of lip movements.

Labiomancy, lipreading.

Labium, lip.

Labor, the process by which a child is delivered from his mother's body. Preparations for labor go on all during pregnancy. The muscles of the uterus tighten and relax. This process of tightening and then relaxing is called a contraction. When labor begins, the contractions of the uterus become more and more frequent and intense. At first these contractions are fifteen or more minutes apart. The time between them gets shorter and shorter as labor progresses. During pregnancy, the cervix (the narrow end of the uterus) softens and relaxes. By the time labor begins, it is thin and has opened to about one half to three quarters of an inch. A small amount of mucus is usually present in this opening as a sort of plug. As the baby is pushed against the cervix by the strong contractions of the uterus, this opening gradually gets larger until it is finally about four inches wide— big enough for the baby to pass through. As the cervix opens, the mucus plug comes loose and is discharged through the vagina. This usually means that labor will begin soon.
A sudden rush of water from the vagina means that the bag of waters surrounding the baby has broken. This may happen at the beginning of labor or not until just before the baby is born. Labor is divided into three stages. In the first stage, the contractions of the uterus stretch the opening at its lower end, the cervix. This allows the baby to move into the birth canal. In the second stage, the baby passes down through the birth canal and out through the vaginal opening. In the third stage, the placenta and membranes (the afterbirth) are loosened and expelled.

Labor, Artificial, induced labor.

Labor, Induced, labor brought on by extraneous means.

Labor Pains, pains produced by the contractions of the womb during labor.

Laboratory, place for testing and experimental work.

Labrum, edge; lip.

Labyrinth, internal ear.

Lac, milk.

Lacerate, to tear.

Laceration, a wound that is torn, rather than cut. Lacerations have ragged, irregular edges and masses of torn or mashed tissue underneath. These wounds are usually made by blunt rather than sharp objects. A wound made by a dull knife, for instance, is more likely to be a laceration than an incision. Many of the wounds caused by accidents with machinery are lacerations, although they are often complicated by crushing of the tissues as well. These wounds, in which the blood vessels are torn or mashed, do not bleed as freely as wounds produced by sharp cutting edges. Lacerations are frequently contaminated with dirt, grease, or other foreign matter that is ground into the tissues; they are therefore very likely to become infected.

Lacertus, muscular portion of the arm.

Lacrimal, pertaining to tears.

Lacrimation, secretion of tears from the eye.

Lactation, the production of milk in the breasts. True milk is not released for at least three days after the birth of a baby. Colostrum, the liquid secreted by the breasts during the first few days, is rich in protein and nourishes the baby until the milk is formed.

Lacteal, relating to milk.

Lactescence, resembling milk.

Lactic Acid, an acid normal to the blood and connected with muscle fatigue.

Lactiferous, conveying milk.

Lactifuge, agent which stops milk secretion.

Lactigenous, producing milk.

Lactin, lactose; a sugar.

Lactinated, containing milk sugar.

Lactoglobulin, protein found in milk.

Lactolin, condensed milk.

Lactose, milk sugar.

Lactotherapy, treatment by milk diet.

Lacuna, small space; pit.

Lag, time between application of a stimulus and the response.

La Grippe, influenza.

Laity, non professional public.

Lake, small fluid cavity.

Laliatry, babbling.

Lalopathy, any speech disorder.

Lambdacism, inability to pronounce the l sound.

Lameness, limping or abnormal walk.

Lamina, thin layer or membrane.

Laminated, in layers.

Lancet, short, double-edged, puncturing knife.

Languor, weariness; exhaustion.

Lanolin, wool fat used in ointments and cosmetics.

Lanugo, fine hair which covers a baby before birth.

Lapactic, purgative.

Laparotomy, surgical incision into the abdominal cavity.

Lapis, stone.

Larva, first stage of an insect from the egg.

Larvate, hidden.

Larvicide, agent which kills larvae.

Laryngectomy, the surgical removal of the larynx. After this operation is performed, most patients can learn to speak again through a technique known as esophageal speech. This substitute speech is produced by expelling swallowed air from the esophagus. A well-trained and practical esophageal voice produces intelligible speech of surprisingly good quality. There are mechanical devices available for those patients who are unable to learn to use this type of speech.

Laryngismus, muscular spasm of the voice box.

Laryngitic, due to laryngitis.

Laryngitis, an inflammation of the larynx (voice box). The primary symptoms of laryngitis are hoarseness and a changed (usually strained sounding) voice. Other symptoms may be a tickling in the throat, a sore throat, and a cough. Laryngitis can be caused by a number of factors. It may follow an infection in the respiratory tract, or it may be a part of another disease such as syphilis or measles. Laryngitis may also be caused by abusing the voice, excessive smoking, breathing unclean air, etc. Additionally, laryngitis can be a symptom of a tumor.

Laryngology, study of the voice box.

Larynx, voice box; the passageway connecting the pharynx and trachea (windpipe).

The larynx is shaped like a tube. It has nine cartilages. One of these, the epiglottis, is responsible for covering the opening of the larynx when the mouth is in the process of swallowing. This closing or lid action prevents foreign material from entering the larynx and eventually reaching the lungs.

There are two pairs of folds in the larynx, but only the vocal folds (also called the true vocal cords) are involved in the production of vocal sound. The area between the vocal folds is known as the glottis.

Sound is produced when air, passing up out of the lungs through the glottis, causes a vibration in the vocal folds. The vibration is controlled by the degree of tension in the folds. A whisper requires less tension than a shout does.

Lassa Fever, a viral infection found in West Africa. Lassa fever causes very high fevers (up to 107°) and severe muscular pain. The fatality rate is high, because the virus kills faster than the body can defend itself.

Latent, hidden.

Lateral, pertaining to the side.

Latrine, public toilet.

Lattissimus, widest.

Lattissimus Dorsi, back muscle.

Latus, Lata, Latum, broad.

Laudable, healthy, normal.

Laughing Gas, nitrous oxide.

Laudanum, tincture of opium.

Lavage, cleansing out an organ.

Lax, without tension.

Laxative, substance when taken helps to evacuate the bowels.

Lazaretto, quarantine station, place for treatment of contagious diseases.

Lead Poisoning, a disease caused by the ingestion of substances containing lead. Studies indicate that children between one and three years of age are the most common victims, although older children also get the disease. Lead poisoning results in damage to the nervous system. The degree of damage is related to the amount and duration of exposure to lead. Once a child has the disease, unless his environment is changed, chances are very high that he will again be a victim. Lead poisoning is caused by consumption over a period of time (three to six months) of paint or plaster containing lead. The condition is frequently associated with pica, which is an abnormal appetite for nonedible substances. In the early stages, the existence of lead poisoning is often without marked symptoms. There may be vague, nonspecific symptoms common in children, such as stomach pain, constipation, vomiting, irritability, and twitching. Unless a high level of suspicion for lead poisoning exists in the physician's mind, the diagnosis may not be recognized. As the disease progresses, the symptoms become stronger, and an elevated amount of lead is found in the blood and urine.

Lean, emaciated; thin.

Lechery, lewdness.

Lechopyra, puerperal fever; child birth fever.

Leech, blood sucking water worm.

Left-Handedness, tendency to use the left hand.

Leg, lower extremity; part of the body from the knee to the ankle.

Leiphemia, thinness of the blood.

Leitrichous, having smooth straight hair.

Lemic, pertaining to any epidemic disease.

Lemology, study of epidemic diseases.

Lemostenosis, stricture of the esophagus.

Lens, magnifying glass; transparent, egg-shaped body behind the pupil of the eye.

Lenticular, lens-shaped.

Lenti-form, lens-shaped.

Lentigo, freckle.

Lentitis, inflammation of the eye lens.

Leper, one afflicted with leprosy.

Lepra, leprosy.

Leprology, study of leprosy.

Leprosarium, place for the care of lepers.

Leprosy, an infectious disease caused by the microorganism *Mycobacterium leprae.* It is not very contagious—only an insignificant percentage of the people who have spent their lives working with leprosy patients have ever contracted it. The method by which it is transmitted is not known.

There are two major types of leprosy: nodular and neural. In nodular leprosy there are masses of nodules that cause distortions in other tissues. In neural leprosy the nerves are affected, frequently producing a numbness and loss of feeling in the affected area; this in turn can result in loss of tissue and bone. The prognosis for patients with leprosy depends to a certain extent on the type of leprosy—patients with neural leprosy generally respond better to treatment than do patients with nodular leprosy.

The treatment for leprosy is primarily chemotherapy (treatment by drugs). The sulfone-class drugs are used with good results for many patients, although it may take up to five years to effect a cure in some types of leprosy. Another drug in use is dapsone.

Leprous, afflicted with leprosy.

Leptodermic, having a thin skin.

Leptophonia, having a feeble voice.

Leptospirosis, a bacterial infection spread to man from animals.

Animal carriers of the leptospirosis bacteria include: cattle, swine, sheep, goats, horses, mules, dogs, cats, foxes, skunks, racoons, wildcats, mongooses, rats, mice, and bats. Leptospirosis bacteria infect the kidneys of animals and are shed through their urine. People can get the disease by swimming in water or walking on moist soil that contains the infected urine. Most frequently, however, people get the disease either by handling a sick animal or by handling the kidney and other infected tissues of an animal that has had leptospirosis. This is why the disease is most prevalent among farmers and other workers who handle animals and animal products. The leptospirosis organism enters the human body through the nose, mouth, eyes, or through a break in the skin. The onset of the disease is sudden, with fever, headache, chills, muscle pains, and sometimes nausea and vomiting. Jaundice, skin rashes, blood in the urine, and a stiff neck are other common symptoms. Because of the numerous and varied symptoms, it is sometimes hard to distinguish this disease from other diseases, including non-paralytic polio, mumps, meningitis, typhoid fever, undulant fever, and influenza. Most cases are quite mild, and the patient recovers in one to two weeks. When the infection is severe, however, the kidney, liver, or heart may be damaged, and death can result.

Leresis, talkativeness in old age.

Lesbianism, homosexuality between women.

Lesion, wound; injury; tumor.

Lethal, fatal; morbid.

Lethargy, marked lack of energy; stupor.

Leucotomy, brain operation used in treatment of some mental disorders.

Leukemia, a fatal disease of the organs that manufacture blood, such as the lymph glands and bone marrow. Normally, these organs manufacture only as many white and red blood cells as the body needs. In leukemia this blood formation gets out of control and there is a tremendous overproduction of white cells. The white cells do not mature, and they are not able to fight infection. The number of red cells is reduced, and the patient becomes anemic. The blood does not clot properly. Patients may thus die from infection, from hemorrhage, or from damage to vital organs. The abnormal cells seen in leukemia resemble cancer cells in appearance and behavior. However, in leukemia the cells are present in the bone marrow and, in the majority of cases, in the blood, as well as in the tissues of the body. In other forms of cancer, the abnormal cells grow in the tissues only. Leukemia can develop at any age. Scientists believe that several factors are involved in the development of leukemia. Recent studies show that radiation can produce the disease. Leukemia can be chronic, acute, or subacute. There are two kinds of chronic leukemia. One begins in the bone marrow and the other in the lymphatic system. The bone-marrow type occurs most often in people thirty-five to forty-five years of age. The lymphatic type is found most frequently in those forty-five to fifty-four years of age. Chronic leukemia affects more men than women. It rarely occurs in children. Chronic leukemia develops slowly, without warning. Many cases are discovered accidentally during examination for some other condition. Even after changes in the blood are noticed, several years may pass before significant symptoms appear in the body. One early change is an enlargement of the blood-forming organs, such as the spleen. As the spleen gets bigger, the patient may feel a sense of fullness or pain in the upper left side of the abdomen. Other symptoms may be sweating, skin eruptions, anemia, hemorrhages, nervousness, and loss of weight. Acute leukemia most often affects children. It usually begins suddenly and progresses rapidly, often with a sore throat or other symptoms of a cold. The glands, spleen, and liver may enlarge rapidly. The child usually becomes pale and bruises easily. However, the beginning of acute leukemia can also develop slowly. In these cases pallor and bone pain are the main symptoms. Without treatment the patient lives only a short time—a few weeks or months. Subacute leukemia has some of the characteristics of both chronic and acute leukemia. The course it follows is harder to predict. Positive diagnosis of leukemia is made by microscopic study of the blood and bone marrow.

Leukoblast, immature white blood cell.

Leukocytes, white blood cells.

Leukocythemia, leukemia.

Leukocytolysis, destruction of white blood cells.

Leukocytosis, increase in the number of white blood cells.

Leukodermia, a condition in which there is a loss of skin pigment in certain areas of the body. The absence of pigment causes patches of very white skin.

Leukopenia, decreased number of white blood cells.

Leukoplakia, white, thickened patches which appear on the skin following chronic irritation.

Leukorrhea, whitish discharge from the womb.

Leukosis, abnormal pallor.

Leukous, white.

Levarterenol, one of the normal secretions of the adrenal glands.

Levoduction, movement of an eye toward the left.

Levorotation, turning to the left.

Libidinous, characterized by lewdness.

Libido, the instinctual energy of life, usually sexual energy.

Lichen, any form of skin disease.

Lichenification, thickening and hardening of the skin.

Licorice, dried root used in medication.

Lid, eyelid.

Lien, spleen.

Lienal, pertaining to the spleen.

Lienectomy, surgical removal of the spleen.

Lienitis, inflammation of the spleen.

Lientery, diarrhea with evacuation of undigested food.

Life, state of being alive.

Ligaments, fibrous bands that hold bones together in the region of a joint.

Ligamentous, pertaining to a ligament.

Ligature, thread for tying off vessels; binding or tying.

Lightening, dropping of the head of the developing infant into the mother's pelvis in the first stage of labor.

Limb, arm or leg.

Limbus, rim; border.

Liminal, barely noticeable.

Limitans, limiting.

Lingism, treatment by exercise.

Limp, impediment in walking.

Linctus, thick syrupy medicine.

Lingua, tongue.

Lingual, pertaining to the tongue.

Liniment, an oily substance rubbed into the skin to relieve pain and muscle cramps.

Linoleic Acid, an important component of many of the unsaturated fats. It is widely found in oils from plants. A diet with a high linoleic acid content tends to lower the amount of cholesterol in the blood.

Lip, external soft structure around the mouth.

Liparous, fat.

Lipemia, fat in the blood.

Lipid, fat.

Lipocyte, fat cell.

Lipogenic, producing fat.

Lipoma, fatty tumor, usually benign.

Lipoprotein, a complex of fat and protein molecules.

Liposarcoma, cancerous tumor composed of undeveloped fat cells.

Lip-Reading, understanding speech by watching the movements of the lips.

Listerism, principles and practice of antiseptic and asceptic surgical procedures.

Liquefacient, converting into a liquid.

Liquescent, becoming liquid.

Lisping, substitution of sounds due to a speech defect, e.g., th for s.

Lithiasis, formation of stone in the body, e.g., gallstones.

Lithotomy, an operation to remove a stone from the bladder.

Litmus Paper, a special, chemically prepared piece of paper that is used to test whether substances are acid or base. Acids turn blue litmus paper red; an alkali (base) will turn red litmus paper blue.

Litter, stretcher.

Livedo, discolored patch of skin.

Liver, important organ of body vitally concerned with metabolism, blood clotting and protein manufacture.

Livid, pale, ashen.

Lividity, discoloration.

Lobar, pertaining to a lobe.

Lobe, globular portion of an organ separated by boundaries.

Lobectomy, surgical removal of a lobe of an organ.

Lobites, inflammation of a lobe.

Lobotomy, cutting across of brain tissue.

Lobule, small lobe; part of a lobe.

Lobus, lobe.

Localization, limited to a definite area; determination of the place of infection.

Lochia, postnatal vaginal discharge. As the uterus grows smaller, clots of blood and tissue flow quite freely and contain a good deal of blood. The flow gradually subsides. At the end of the first week it has changed in color from bright red to dark red or brown. At the end of the second week it may be yellow or white, but it is not unusual for the dark discharge to persist for a while longer. Although this discharge from the vagina is often called menstruation, it is not.

Lochiopyra, puerperal fever.

Lock Jaw, tetanus.

Locomotion, movement from place to place.

Loculpus, small space; cavity.

Locus, place; site.

Logamnesia, inability to recall words.

Logokophosis, word deafness.

Logopathy, any speech disorder of central origin.

Logopedia, study and treatment of speech defects.

Loin, portion of back between thorax and pelvis.

Longevity, long life.

Longsightedness, farsightedness.

Lordosis, an abnormal curvature of the spine with the convexity towards the front.

Lotio, lotion.

Lotion, liquid substance for washing a part.

Loupe, convex lens.

Louse, parasite that transmits diseases.
Three kinds of lice (the head louse, the body louse, and the pubic or crab louse) infest the human body. The names of the three types indicate the areas of the body on which each is usually found. Head and body lice look alike, but their habits are different. Lack of personal cleanliness is a common cause of infestation; however, any child or adult may inadvertently acquire an infestation by contact with infested people or articles. While the lice themselves seldom cause serious trouble, the scratching they induce sometimes results in skin lesions and infections.

Loxia, wry neck.

Loxotic, slanting.

Loxotomy, oblique amputation.

Lozenge, soothing, medicated solid to be held in the mouth until it dissolves.

LSD, legally classed as a hallucinogen, a mind-affecting drug, LSD is noted mainly for producing strong and bizarre mental reactions in people and striking distortions in their physical senses—what and how they see, touch, smell, and hear.
Just how LSD works in the body is not yet known. It seems to affect the levels of certain chemicals in the

brain and to produce changes in the brain's electrical activity. Animal experiments with LSD suggest that the brain's normal filtering and screening-out process becomes blocked, causing it to become flooded with unselected sights and sounds. Studies of chronic LSD users indicate that they continue to suffer from an overload of stimulation to their senses. Researchers believe this may explain the regular user's inability to think clearly and to concentrate on a goal.

Lubb-Dupp, vocal interpretation of heart sounds.

Lubricant, an agent which makes smooth.

Lucid, clear.

Lucipetal, attracted by bright light.

Lues, syphilis.

Lumbago, backache in the loin region.

Lumbar, pertaining to the loin.

Lumbodynia, lumbago.

Lumen, space within a tube.

Luminal, sedative; phenobarbital.

Lunacy, mental illness.

Lunatic, insane person.

Lungs, two cone-shaped bodies responsible for providing the body with air and with discharging certain waste products. The lungs are soft, spongy, and elastic. The outside of each lung is covered by a closed sac called the pleura. The inner part of the lungs communicates freely with the outside air through the windpipe. The outside of the lungs is protected from air pressure by the walls of the chest cavity, creating a lessened pressure within the enveloping lung sac. The air pressure within the lungs expands them until they fill almost the entire chest cavity. If any air gets through the chest wall, or if the lung is punctured so that air from the outside can communicate with the pleural sac, the lungs shrink because the air pressure is equalized outside and inside the chest cavity. The lungs are not equal in size. The right lung has three lobes, and the left lung has two lobes. These lobes are closed systems, so that any one lobe can be removed without damage to the remaining lobes. In passing to and from the lungs, air passes through the nose, throat, and the windpipe (trachea). In the nose the air is warmed and moistened. By means of the moist hairs and the moist mucous membrane of the nose, much of the dust is filtered out of inhaled air. Moreover, the sense of smell, which warns of the presence of some types of harmful gases, is situated in the nose. By the time air reaches the lungs it is much safer for them. Large bronchial tubes (bronchi) leading from the windpipe carry the air that has been breathed in through the mouth and nose. These large tubes divide into smaller and smaller ones (bronchioles) until they are the size of fine threads. At the end of each small tube there is a cluster of tiny air sacs called alveoli. These air cells resemble a bunch of grapes, except they are many times smaller. Around each air cell, which has very thin walls, is a fine network of small blood vessels or capillaries. The blood in these capillaries releases carbon dioxide and other waste matter brought from tissue activity all over the body. This takes place through the thin air-cell wall. In exchange, the blood takes on a supply of oxygen from the air breathed into the air cells. The discarded carbon dioxide and waste matter are removed from the air cells in the air that is breathed out of the lungs. This process is repeated about sixteen times every minute.

Lunula, pale crescent at root of nail.

Lupiform, resembling lupus.

Lupous, pertaining to lupus.

Lupus, disease of unknown origin affecting skin and vital organs.

Lusus Natural, freak of nature.

Luxation, dislocation.

Luxus, excess.

Lying-in, puerperal state; child-bed.

Lymph, special functioning fluid that flows through specific vessels, passing through the filter of the lymph glands before entering the blood stream.

Lymphadentis, inflammation of a lymph gland.

Lymphatic, relating to lymph or a vessel through which it flows.

Lymph System, a circulatory system of vessels, spaces, and nodes. The lymph system carries lymph, the almost-colorless fluid that bathes the body's cells. The lymph nodes are small glands that act as filters for the lymph system. They remove bacteria, etc., from the lymph as it passes through the nodes. These nodes produce white blood cells and antibodies to help the body defend against infection. Lymph nodes are scattered throughout the body in clumps. The principal areas are the hand, neck, face, armpits, chest, abdomen, pelvic region, groin, and legs. In addition to the lymph nodes, the lymph system also includes three other lymph organs. These organs are the spleen, the tonsils, and the thymus. Part of the function of the spleen is to produce white blood cells and to help the lymph nodes act as a filter. The tonsils and the thymus also manufacture white blood cells.

Lysemia, disintegration of the blood.

Lysis, gradual disappearance of a disease.

Lyssa, rabies.

Lyssoid, resembling rabies.

Maceration, soften in a fluid.

Machonnement, chewing motion.

Macies, wasting.

Macrobiosis, longevity.

Macrocephalus, having an unusually large head.

Macrocyte, large red blood cell.

Macrodont, having large teeth.

Macropodia, unusually large feet.

Macroscopic, visible to the naked eye.

Macrosonia, gigantism.

Macula, pigmented spot on the skin, spot in the retina.

Maculate, spotted.

Mad, insane; angry.

Madarosis, loss of eyelashes or eyebrows.

Madescent, damp.

Madura Foot, disease of the foot caused by a fungus infection.

Maduromycosis, an infection that is caused by fungus. Maduromycosis usually affects the foot but may also be found in the hand and other body parts. The fungus generally enters the body through a wound. Maduromycosis is most frequently found in warm climates. The fungus causes lesions and pus to form. The pus is discharged through dead tissue. If untreated, maduromycosis will destroy tissue and bone. Some forms of this disease, caused by specific molds, are treatable with penicillin and sulfonamides. However, other types will not respond to drugs, and in those cases the only treatment is amputation of the affected part. An untreated case of maduromycosis can lead to death as a result of secondary infections.

Maggot, worm.

Magnesium, a mineral that is essential to the proper functioning of the body. Large amounts are found in the bones and the teeth. Among other functions, it plays an indispensable role in the body's use of food for energy. Magnesium is found in goodly amounts in nuts, whole-grain products, dry beans, dry peas, and dark-green vegetables.

Maidenhead, hymen.

Maidism, pellagra.

Maieutics, obstetrics.

Maim, injure, disable.

Main, hand.

Main Succulente, edema of the hands.

Mal, sickness; pain; disease.

Mala, cheek; cheekbone.

Malabsorptive Disease, an inability to digest and absorb food properly.

Malacosarcosis, softness of muscle tissue.

Malacosteon, softening of the bones.

Malacostic, soft.

Malady, illness.

Malaise, uneasiness, indisposition.

Malar, pertaining to the cheek or cheek bone.

Malaria, acute, febrile, infectious disease caused by the presence of parasitic organisms in the red blood cells. The process by which malaria is transmitted requires one person already infected with malaria, one or more healthy people, and a female *Anopheles* mosquito. The cycle begins when this female mosquito bites the person who has malaria. The blood that is sucked into the mosquito's body contains the malaria parasites. The parasites develop into the infective stage within the insect's body. These parasites will develop over a two-week period. After this time any person the mosquito bites will become infected. This is because the mosquito injects the infective parasites at the same time it is sucking blood out of the person. About ten days to two weeks (although the incubation period can vary more than that) after being bitten, the infected person begins to exhibit the symptoms of malaria. The classic symptoms are a cycle of fever and chills, but they usually also include headache and nausea. Different varieties of malaria have different cycles. In one kind, the fever and chills occur every other day; in another type, they appear every third day; and others have different patterns.

Malariologist, specialist in malaria.

Malassimilation, defective assimilation.

Malaxation, kneading motion in massage.

Male, masculine; fertilizing member of the sex.

Malformation, deformity, an abnormal development.

Malignant, poisonous, threatening life.

Malignant Hypertension, a severe form of high blood pressure that runs a rapid course. It causes damage to the blood vessel walls in the kidneys, eyes, etc.

Malingerer, one who fakes illness and pretends to be suffering.

Malleolus, an extension of bone having the shape of a hammerhead on either side of the ankle joint.

Malleus, one of the three tiny, linked bones in the middle ear. The malleus (also called the hammer) is the outer bone that is attached to the eardrum. The vibrations of the eardrum are passed on to the malleus. At the other end of the malleus is the second of the three middle ear bones, the incus. The vibrations of the malleus are moved along to the incus.

Malnutrition, an impairment or risk of impairment to physical and mental health caused by failure to meet nutritional requirements. Malnutrition is the result of either the consumption of an insufficient quantity of food or of one or more essential nutrients. It may also be caused by faulty absorption or utilization of nutrients owing to physical or emotional causes. In this country the most usual consequence of deficient diet is general undernutrition of a rather mild degree. As a rule, this is caused by a diet that is low in a number of essentials, and it develops when a person eats one food to excess and gets too little of other foods. The amount of iron, calcium, and other minerals may all be insufficient, or the diet may furnish insufficient vitamins. The consumption of protein may be inadequate in quantity, or in quality, or in both for the best growth of muscles and other tissues. Malnutrition may also occur when the total food intake is not enough to supply the energy needed for bodily activities. A chronic disease or some particular physical defect may interfere with nutrition. Poor mental health, or simply unhappiness, may also be a factor. Such conditions may prevent a person from eating as much as he should or may interfere with his ability to utilize what he does eat. These situations usually result in a combination of mild symptoms of various diseases and in a general lack of well-being.

Malocclusion, a condition in which the upper and lower teeth do not meet evenly, resulting in an incorrect bite.

Malposition, abnormal position of any organ or part.

Malpractice, improper medical care due to carelessness or ignorance of the doctor.

Malpresentation, faulty fetal presentation.

Malum, disease.

Malunion, a condition in which a broken bone has healed improperly and the broken edges of the bone are not evenly matched together. Malunion occurs when the broken bone has not been properly set or has not been set at all. The condition is corrected by deliberately breaking the bone again and setting it properly.

Mamma Virilis, male breast.

Mammalgia, breast pain.

Mammary Glands, the breasts.

Mammilla, nipple.

Mammillary, resembling a nipple.

Mammogram, special type of x-ray used to examine the soft tissue of the breast to confirm or rule out the presence of cancer.

Mammose, having unusually large breasts.

Mancinism, left-handedness.

Mandible, lower jawbone.

Mandibular, pertaining to the mandible or lower jaw bone.

Manducation, chewing.

Maneuver, skillful procedure.

Mania, violent passion or desire; extreme excitement.

Maniac, one obsessed by a violent passion or desire.

Manic-Depressive, characterized by alternate excitement and depression.

Manipulation, skillful use of the hands.

Mantle, brain cortex.

Mantoux test, a simple skin test for detecting tuberculosis.

Manual, pertaining to the hands.

Manubrium, handle; top part of the breastbone.

Manus, hand.

Maple Syrup Urine Disease, a defect in the metabolism of certain protein builders. This causes a "maple syrup" odor to urine; seizures; mental retardation; and early death. A special diet may be successful for prevention.

Marasmic, pertaining to marasmus.

Marasmus, progressive wasting in infants without an obvious cause.

Mareo, seasickness.

Margo, pl., **Margines,** border, margin.

Marihuana, a dried plant material from the Indian hemp plant *(Cannabis sativa)*. The plant grows wild in many parts of the world, including the United States, and is frequently cultivated for its commercial value in the production of fiber for rope, in birdseed, and for other purposes. In its drug use it is known by such names as "pot," "grass," "weed," "Mary Jane," and many others. For use as a drug, the leaves and flowering tops of the plant are dried and crushed or broken into small fragments which are then typically rolled into thin, homemade cigarettes, often called "joints." It may also be smoked in small pipes and is occasionally incorporated into food and eaten. The smoke smells like burning rope or alfalfa. Because of its distinctive odor, users sometimes burn incense to mask the smell. Hashish ("hash") is the potent, dark-brown resin that is collected from the tops of high-quality cannabis. Because of the high concentration of resin, it is often five to six times stronger than the usual marihuana, although the active drug ingredients are the same. Basically, it is a much more concentrated form of the drug. When smoked, marihuana quickly enters the bloodstream and within minutes begins to affect the user's mood and thinking. The exact mechanisms of action and the alterations of cerebral metabolism are not well understood. Extensive research is currently underway to provide this basic information. Because it can cause hallucinations if used in very high doses, marihuana is technically classified as a mild hallucinogen.

Mark, spot; blemish.

Marrow, the spongy, porous material found in the center of a bone. Until adulthood, bone marrow is red because it is actively producing red blood cells. When adulthood has been reached and there is no further growth, many bones no longer produce red blood cells. These bones then have a yellow bone marrow, which is largely composed of fat. However, because red blood cells constantly wear out and must be replaced, some of the bones in the body continue to have red bone marrow.

Marsh Fever, malarial fever.

Marsupium, pouch.

Masculation, having male characteristics.

Masculine, pertaining to the male.

Masculinization, acquisition of male secondary sex characteristics by the female.

Masochism, sexual pleasure derived from pain.

Masochist, one who derives pleasure from pain.

Massage, treatment of disease of the tissues.

Masseur, man who massages.

Masseuse, woman who massages.

Mastadenitis, mammary gland inflammation.

Mastadenoma, breast tumor.

Mastalgia, pain in the breast.

Mastauxe, breast enlargement.

Mastectomy, surgical removal of the breast.

Mastication, the process of chewing food to reduce it to the point where it can be comfortably swallowed. Mastication is the first of the digestive processes.

Mastitis, inflammation of the breasts.

Mastodynia, pain in the breast.

Mastoid, bone situated behind the ear; nipple-shaped.

Mastoidectomy, surgical destruction of the cells in the mastoid.

Mastology, study of the breasts.

Mastoncus, breast tumor, swelling.

Masturbation, self-stimulation of the sex organs.

Materia, material; substance.

Materia Medica, pharmacology.

Maternal, pertaining to the mother.

Matrix, pl., **Matrices,** uterus, generative structure.

Maturation, achieving maturity.

Mature, fully developed.

Maxilla, bone of the upper jaw.

Maxillofacial, pertaining to the lower half of the face.

M.B., Bachelor of Medicine.

M.D., Doctor of Medicine.

Mean, average.

Measles, an infectious viral disease marked by fever, a rash of pink spots, redness of the eyes and mild bronchitis. The virus that causes measles is found in the secretions of the nose and throat of infected persons who discharge virus particles into the air when they talk, sneeze, or cough. People become infected by inhaling these virus particles. It is also possible to become infected with the virus by touching articles that have been in recent contact with an infected person's nose or mouth, such as handkerchiefs or clothes. Measles can be dangerous because of the complications that can follow it. These include bronchopneumonia, middle-ear infection, and encephalitis. The encephalitis that occurs in about one out of every one thousand cases of measles often causes permanent brain damage, resulting in mental retardation

Measles-German, an acute viral fever which is like a mild attack of measles, running a shorter course.

Meatus, opening; passage.

Mecamylamine Hydrochloride, a drug that blocks the transmission of nerve impulses at the nerve centers.

Meconium, opium; first feces of the newborn.

Medi- (prefix), middle.

Medial, pertaining to the middle.

Median, located in the middle.

Mediastinum, a term used to indicate the area between the lungs. It contains the heart, trachea, esophagus, etc.

Medicable, receptive to cure.

Medical, pertaining to medicine.

Medical Examiner, an official whose duty it is to determine cause of death in questionable cases.

Medical Jurisprudence, medicine and its relation to law.

Medicament, medicinal substance.

Medication, giving of remedies; medicinal agent.

Medicinal, of a curative nature.

Medicine, art and science of healing.

Medicolegal, pertaining to medical jurisprudence.

Medicus, doctor.

Medulla, marrow.

Medulla Oblongata, cone-shaped part of the nervous system which is at the junction between the spinal cord and the brain.

Medullary, pertaining to a medulla.

Medullispinal, pertaining to the spinal cord.

Medullitis, inflammation of marrow.

Megacephalic, having an unusually large head.

Magalgia, acute pain.

Megalocornea, bulging of the cornea.

Megalogastria, enlargement of the stomach.

Megalohepatia, enlargement of the liver.

Megalomania, delusions of personal grandeur.

Megalomelia, unusual largeness of the limbs.

Megarectum, enlargement of the rectum.

Megrim, migraine.

Meibomian Glands, glands located near the upper and lower eyelids.

Mel, honey.

Melaena, black vomit.

Melalgia, pain in the extremities.

Melancholia, depression and self pity.

Melanin, black or dark-brown pigment.

Melanoglossia, black tongue.

Melanoma, tumor arising from a pigmented mole.

Melanopathy, excessive skin pigmentation.

Melanosis, deposits of black pigment found in various parts of the body.

Melasma, dark pigmentation.

Melena, very dark bowel movements, an indication of internal bleeding.

Melitemia, excess blood sugar.

Melitis, inflammation of cheek.

Mellite, honey preparation.

Membrana, membrane.

Membrane, thin layer of tissue covering or dividing an organ.

Membranoid, resembling a membrane.

Membrum, body; part; organ.

Memory, recall of past experience.

Menacme, years of menstrual activity in a woman's life.

Menarche, onset of the menstrual period.

Meniere's Disease, a disease of the organs of balance in the inner ear in which there is deafness and sudden attacks of extreme giddiness, vomiting and loss of balance.

Meninges, three layered membranes that cover and protect the brain and the spinal cord. The three layers are: the dura mater, the arachnoid and the pia mater. The dura mater is the outermost layer and is the toughest of the three membranes. Beneath the dura mater is the arachnoid, so named because it resembles a spider's web. Beneath the arachnoid, and closest to the brain, is the pia mater, a transparent membrane that actually touches the brain and spinal cord.

Meningioma, tumor arising from membranes covering the brain.

Meningitides, inflammation of the lining membrane of the brain or spinal cord.

Meningitis, inflammation of the lining of the brain and spinal cord with both mental and motor systems usually involved.

It may be caused by any of several bacteria, viruses, or other microscopic organisms. A very serious form is caused by an organism called meningococcus. These bacteria may be present in the body with no effect, or they may cause serious illness. If meningococci reach the brain or spinal cord, they cause severe inflammation or meningitis. Without treatment, this disease is fatal in about half the cases; survivors may be left with disabilities such as deafness and paralysis. Meningitis usually begins suddenly, with severe headache and stiffness and pains in the neck, back, and shoulders. Other symptoms are a high fever and often nausea and vomiting. A skin rash of tiny, bright-red spots frequently occurs. If these conditions appear, a physician should be consulted, because prompt treatment is essential. A diagnosis of meningitis is confirmed by inserting a needle into the spinal column to withdraw fluid. This fluid is then analyzed.

Antibiotics and sulfa drugs are effective in most cases of meningococcal meningitis. With early treatment, most patients get well quickly. A few deaths result from an overwhelming infection that defies even prompt treatment.

Meningomalacia, softening of a membrane.

Meningopathy, any disease of the meninges.

Meninx, see meninges.

Meniscus, crescent-shaped piece of gristle usually found in the knee joint.

Menolipsis, temporary absence of menstruation.

Menopause, the end of menstrual periods and, therefore, the end of childbearing years. It is also called the climacteric or "change of life." The menopause usually occurs when a woman is between forty and fifty. It can occur earlier or later. It starts gradually and is recognized by the change in menstruation. The monthly flow becomes smaller in amount, then irregular, and finally ceases. Often, the time between periods becomes longer and longer—there may be a lapse of several months between them. Before and during these changes in the monthly periods, certain symptoms may appear; e.g., hot or warm flushes, dizziness, weakness, nervousness, and insomnia. Many women have very mild symptoms; some have none at all; with a few, the discomfort is very severe. The symptoms are caused by the disappearance of the female sex hormone that the ovaries produce. The same symptoms occur when the ovaries are removed surgically because of disease (surgical menopause). After a period of time ranging from a few months to a year or two, the body adjusts itself, and the symptoms disappear. While this adjustment is taking place, hot flushes, etc., can appear. The menopause is not a complete change of life. The normal sex urges remain, and women retain their usual reaction to sex long after the menopause. Medical treatment can be very successful in relieving symptoms of menopause. Medical care can help to correct nervousness and low spirits that often go along with menopause. Mental depression is not unusual at this time.

Menorrhagia, excessive bleeding during the monthly period.

Menorrhea, normal menstruation; profuse menstruation.

Menoschesis, suppression of menstruation.

Menostaxis, prolonged menstruation.

Menses, menstruation.

Menstruation, the periodic shedding of the lining of the uterus. About every twenty-eight days, midway between two menstrual cycles, changes take place in both the ovaries and the uterus. An ovary prepares to release one of its ova. At the same time, the lining of the uterus starts to grow. Tiny glands and blood vessels appear in the top half of this lining, and the whole of it becomes soft and velvety. About fourteen days before the menstrual flow, a single ovum leaves one of the ovaries, stops for twenty-four hours at the entrance to a fallopian tube, then goes on through the tube into the uterus. If conception does not take place, the lining of the uterus then gradually stops growing and comes loose. As it loosens, the blood vessels that come away with it begin to bleed. This causes the menstrual flow of blood, which lasts several days. It carries away the unused top layer of the lining of the uterus and any other waste materials that may be present. As soon as this first menstrual period ends, preparation for another one begins. This cycle repeats itself, except during pregnancy, until the menopause.

Mensuration, measuring.

Mental, pertaining to the mind; pertaining to the chin.

Mental Illness, a mental or emotional disorder strong enough to interfere in a major or minor way with daily living.

Mental disorders can be classified under four major headings: psychoses, neuroses, personality or character disorders, and psychosomatic diseases.

Psychoses (which the term "insanity" usually refers to) are generally characterized by strange feelings and behavior and by a distortion of reality. Psychoses are the most severe forms of mental illness.

The neuroses are less severe emotional disturbances, although in some cases thinking and judgment may be impaired. The trouble is mostly in the way a neurotic person feels—and often he feels very uncomfortable. Neurotics may be continually bothered by feelings of anxiety or depression, which use up their energies and fill them with nameless dread.

Character or personality disorders are difficulties in adjustment that show themselves in the kind of disturbed behavior that is seen in the drug addict, the chronic alcoholic, or the delinquent. Usually the person with a character disorder does not feel great anxiety or guilt about his behavior, whereas most other emotionally ill persons with the same symptoms do. He behaves very much as if he does not care about the standards of conduct or achievement that are important to most people in our society. Irresponsibility and immaturity are often indications of this type of disorder.

Psychosomatic diseases are those ailments in which the symptoms are primarily physical, although there may be a large emotional component.

Mental Retardation, a condition of inadequately developed intelligence that significantly impairs the ability to learn and to adapt to the demands of society. Mental retardation is present at birth or develops during childhood and usually continues throughout life. More than two hundred specific causes of mental retardation have been identified. In approximately twenty to twenty-five percent of cases the cause is known. Among the known biological factors are hereditary factors, infections, nutritional deficiencies or toxic substances in the mother's system during pregnancy, and injuries. Lack of a healthful environment, including motivation, stimulation, and opportunity, is a large factor for many children.

Some mentally retarded children are behind in various stages of their development such as sitting up, crawling, walking, and talking. Some are born with a combination of physical signs such as those in mongolism (Down's syndrome), which usually makes possible a diagnosis at birth. Other babies, born normal, develop jaundice in the first days of life. This warns the doctor that mental retardation may be threatening unless immediate steps are taken. A child with the enlarged head of hydrocephalus (excess fluid inside the skull) is in danger of mental retardation. Other retarded children are, in all obvious ways, physically healthy and normal. Their mental retardation may not even be suspected until they enter school and cannot keep up with normal children. The degree of mental retardation may range from mild to profound. In severe cases the condition is usually recognizable very early; when slight, it may require several years of observation to make the proper diagnosis. In terms of physical appearance, seventy-five percent of the retarded have the same characteristics as the rest of the population. On this basis alone only twenty-five percent are detectable through differences in head size, small stature, small hands, or slanted eyes. The overriding symptom of mental retardation is that the individual does not adapt or achieve in the same manner or degree as his contemporaries. Mental retardation is classified on the basis of measured intelligence and adaptive behavior.

Mentum, chin.

Mephitic, noxious; foul.

Meralgia, thigh pain.

Mercurial Diuretic, one of various compounds of mercury commonly used to promote the elimination of water and sodium from the body through increased excretion of urine.

Meropia, partial blindness.

Merotomy, cutting into sections.

Mesiad, toward the center.

Mesial, located in the middle.

Mesmerism, hypnotism.

Metabolism, the building-up and breaking-down processes of the body as a whole.

Metabolism, Basal, minimum amount of energy necessary to maintain life when the body is at complete rest.

Metacarpus, five bones in the palm of the hand.

Metachrosis, change of color.

Metachysis, blood transfusion.

Metacyesis, extrauterine pregnancy.

Metallophobia, extreme fear of metallic objects.

Metamorphosis, change of shape or structure.

Metaphase, the second stage in cell division.

Metastasis, movement of bacteria or a disease from one part of the body to another.

Metatarsus, part of the foot between the ankle and the beginning of the toes.

Methadone, a synthetic drug that can be given to a heroin addict to replace heroin. Methadone has the advantage of being less expensive and allowing the addict to maintain a normal life. However, methadone is also an addictive drug.

Methamphetamine, a stimulant, or a drug that stimulates the central nervous system. Methamphetamine is similar to amphetamine, but in many ways it is stronger. While methamphetamine does have important medical uses, it has become a drug of abuse, known as "speed."

Metopagus, twins joined at the forehead.

Metopic, pertaining to the forehead.

Metra, the uterus.

Metralgia, pain in the uterus.

Metrectasia, dilatation of the uterus.

Metritis, inflammation of the uterus.

Metrocarcinoma, cancer of the uterus.

Metrocyte, mother cell.

Metrodynia, pain in the uterus.

Metrology, science of measurements.

Metropathy, any uterine disorder.

Metrorrhagia, vaginal bleeding unrelated to monthly bleeding.

M.F.D., minimum fatal dose.

Miasm, Miasma, foul odor.

Mication, involuntary, rapid winking; fast motion.

Microbe, small, living organism discernible only through a microscope.

Microbicidal, destroying microbes.

Microbiologist, specialist in microbiology.

Microbiology, science dealing with microscopic organisms.

Microcardia, abnormal smallness of the heart.

Microcoria, smallness of the pupil.

Microcyst, tiny cyst.

Microcyte, small red blood corpuscle.

Microglossia, abnormal smallness of the tongue.

Microlesion, very small lesion.

Micromastia, unusual smallness of the breast.

Micronize, reduce to very small particles.

Microorganism, microscopic organism.

Microphallus, abnormal smallness of the penis.

Micropsia, defective vision; seeing things smaller than they are.

Microscope, instrument which enlarges objects for visual examination.

Microscopic, able to be seen only under a microscope.

Microscopy, observation with the microscope.

Micturition, urination.

Midget, one who does not attain full growth; very small person.

Midriff, diaphragm.

Midwife, woman who helps at childbirth.

Midwifery, obstetrics.

Midriasis, enlargement of the pupil of the eye.

Migraine, severe, periodic, onesided headache, usually ac-companied by abdominal distress.

Miliaria, heat rash.

Milieu, environment.

Milk, one of the most important of all foods. Babies begin life on a milk diet because it is so rich in important pro-teins, vitamins, etc. Milk is also important to growing children because of the amount of calcium it provides.

Milphosis, loss of eyebrows or eyelashes.

Minerals, inorganic substances that are essential to the human body. They give strength and rigidity to certain body tissues and help with numerous vital functions. Most of the hard tissues of the human body, such as bones and teeth, are composed in part of mineral ele-ments. In the case of bones and teeth, relatively large amounts of calcium and phosphorus are needed to make up these structures, but the body also needs many other minerals, some in very minute quantities, to carry on its life processes. For instance, in order to function properly, muscles, nerves, and the heart must be constantly nourished by body fluids containing the correct proportion of minerals such as sodium, potas-sium, and calcium. Similarly, red blood cells cannot be formed or function properly unless sufficient iron is supplied to the body. The consumption of small amounts of another mineral, fluorine, during the forma-tive years prevents excessive tooth decay among young children and adolescents and during later life. Al-together, about fifteen different mineral elements are required by the body, and all must be derived from food or drink. The minerals in which diets are most likely to be low, or deficient, are calcium, iron, iodine, and fluorine.

Miocardia, heart contraction.

Miosis, contraction.

Miscarriage, loss of product of conception before age of viability; abortion.

Miscarriages may be caused by factors other than ab-normalities of the egg or infant. They may also be caused by glandular or nutritional problems. Miscar-riage used to be blamed on a fall or a blow to the ab-domen, but doctors now know that this is an exceed-ingly rare cause. The baby is protected within a sac of fluid in the uterus and usually escapes injury even in the event of a serious accident to the mother. Slight bleeding may mean that a miscarriage is only threatening and that the baby may yet be saved. More severe bleeding, especially with cramps, usually means that a miscarriage is actually in progress.

Miscegenation, people of two different races that are married.

Miscible, able to be mixed.

Misogamy, hatred of marriage.

Misopedia, hatred of children.

Mite, tiny insect.

Mitosis, the process of human cell division or reproduction.

Mitral Valve, the heart valve on left side of heart between upper and lower chambers.

Mitral Valvulotomy, an operation to widen the opening in the valve between the upper and lower chambers in the left side of the heart (mitral valve).

Mittelschmerz, pain at time of ovulation.

M.M., mucous membrane.

Mnemonics, improvement of the memory.

Mobile, movable.

Moccasin, poisonous snake.

Modus, method.

Modus Operandi, method of performing an act.

Mogigraphia, writers' cramp.

Mogilalia, speech defect.

Mogitocia, difficult birth.

Moist, damp.

Molar, the teeth that grind food. The first permanent teeth are the four "6-year" molars, one on each side of the upper and lower jaws. Appearing about the sixth year, behind the primary teeth, they are often mistaken for primary teeth. The "6-year" molars are very important. They make it possible for the child to chew during the time the primary teeth are being replaced by permanent teeth. The position of the "6-year" molars largely determines the position of the other permanent teeth, which in turn influence the shape of the jaws and the child's appearance. If the "6-year" molars are lost, the shape of the jaw may be changed, and correction and alignment may later be required. There are three sets of molars. The first set is the "6-year" molars. The second set erupts at the age of twelve or thirteen. The third and final set emerges between the ages of seventeen and twenty-one. These last molars are often referred to as the "wisdom teeth."

Mold, fungus.

Molding, shaping of the fetal head at birth.

Mole, skin growth usually colored and sprouting hair.

Molecule, tiny mass of matter.

Molimen, effort to establish the monthly period.

Mollities, abnormal softening.

Molluscum, chronic skin disease with pulpy bumps.

Monarticular, pertaining to a single joint.

Mongolism, arrest of physical and mental development, with features similar to the Asiatic race.

Moniliasis, fungus infection of various areas of the body, especially mouth, throat, vagina.

Moniliform, beaded.

Monocular, pertaining to or affecting one eye; having a single lens.

Monocular Vision, a condition in which one eye is blind or one eye refuses to register images in coordination with the better eye.

Monocyesis, pregnancy with one fetus.

Monocyte, type of white blood cell.

Monodiplopia, double vision in one eye.

Monogenesis, nonsexual reproduction.

Monogenous, a sexual reproduction.

Monohemerous, lasting only one day.

Monomania, obsession with one subject or idea.

Monomelic, affecting one limb.

Mononucleosis, glandular fever; virus disease in which monocytes are increased beyond normal number, lymph nodes enlarged, sore throat.

Monopathy, disease affecting a single part.

Monoplegia, paralysis of a single group of muscles or one limb.

Monosexual, having characteristics of only one sex.

Mono-unsaturated Fat, a fat so constituted chemically that it is capable of absorbing additional hydrogen but not as much hydrogen as a polyunsaturated fat.

Mood, attitude; state of mind.

Mons, elevated area.

Mons Pubis, Mons Veneris, area over the symphysis pubis in the female.

Monster, abnormally formed fetus.

Monstrosity, state of being a monster.

Monthlies, menses.

Monticulus, protuberance.

Morbid, pertaining to disease; the disease itself.

Morbid Condition, condition of disease.

Morbidity Rate, the ratio of the number of cases of a disease to the number of healthy people in a given population during a specified period of time.
Incidence is the number of new cases of a disease developing in a given population during a specified period of time. Prevalence is the number of cases of a given disease existing in a given population at a specified moment of time.

Morbific, causing disease.

Morbilli, measles.

Morbilliform, like measles.

Morbus, disease.

Morbus Caducus, epilepsy.

Mores, customs.

Morgue, public mortuary.

Moria, foolishness.

Moribund, dying.

Morning Sickness, nausea and vomiting during the early stages of pregnancy.

Moron, one whose mental age is from seven to twelve years.

Morosis, feeblemindedness.

Morphine, drug used as an analgesic and sedative.
Morphine, like all narcotics, is physically addictive. A patient taking morphine over a period of time develops a tolerance for the drug and requires larger and larger doses. There is also a danger of psychological dependency developing in the case of a patient using mor-

phine over a period of time. The size of the dose of morphine determines, to a certain extent, the degree of side effects present. As the level of the dose increases, so does the degree of the side effects. Morphine tends to make the patient drowsy, changes his mood (often to euphoria), produces constipation, and can cause nausea and vomiting.

Morphinism, addiction to morphine.

Mors, death.

Morsus, bite.

Morsus Humanus, human bite.

Mortal, deadly.

Mortise Joint, ankle joint.

Mosquito, blood sucking insect.

Mosquitocide, agent which kills mosquitoes.

Mother, female parent.

Mother's Mark, birthmark.

Motile, able to move.

Motion Sickness, a feeling of nausea that may be accompanied by vomiting and which is caused by motion. Motion sickness presents two problems. The first is the physical problem. Motion sickness is caused by an upset in the delicate balance mechanism of the inner ear. The parts of the inner ear that control balance (the semicircular canals and their appendages) have fluids in them. When the fluid moves, it touches small hairs, which in turn trigger nerve impulses to the brain. When the amount of motion and/or the kind of motion is sufficiently aggravating, the vomiting center of the brain is also triggered.
The second problem associated with motion sickness is a psychological one. The fear of flying can upset the stomach enough to cause motion sickness. Once a person has had motion sickness, whether from physical or psychological factors, he is prone to have motion sickness again. Thus, in addition to being afraid to travel, or actually having a disturbance in the balance mechanism, he also has to cope with his fear of motion sickness.

Mottling, discoloration in various areas.

Mounding, lumping.

Mountain Sickness, condition caused by low air pressure.

Mouth, the first part of the digestive system. The mouth is a cavity consisting of the hard palate and the teeth at the top, the cheeks as the side, the tongue and lower teeth as the floor, and the soft palate extending from the end of the hard palate to the pharynx.

The digestive functions of the mouth are mastication and lubrication. The teeth reduce food to manageable size. Saliva prepares the food to move easily down the rest of the digestive tract.

The mouth, an important part of speech, is also an alternate breathing passage.

M.S., Master of Surgery.

M.T., Medical Technologist.

Muciferous, secreting mucus.

Mucilage, paste.

Mucilaginous, adhesive.

Mucin, main substance of mucus.

Mucopus, mucus mixed with pus.

Mucosa, mucous membrane; lining tissue that produces mucus.

Mucous, pertaining to mucus.

Mucus, a thick, white liquid secreted by mucous glands.

Mulatto, anyone of both Negro and White blood.

Muliebria, female genitalia.

Muliebrity, femininity.

Multi- (prefix), many; much.

Multigravida, pregnant woman who had more than two past pregnancies.

Multipara, woman who has had more than two live children.

Multiple Sclerosis, a chronic, progressive, degenerative disease of the central nervous system.

Multiple sclerosis is not contagious nor is it a mental disease. It is "multiple" in the sense that it produces multiple changes or lesions on the brain and spinal cord, which result in multiple effects in the body. More often multiple sclerosis attacks one area of the nervous system and later, after a period of improvement, the same area again or a different place. It is "sclerotic" because it leaves sclera or scars at the points where demyelination, the loss of the protective covering of the nerves, takes place. For this reason, multiple sclerosis is known as a demyelinating disease. The fatty covering called "myelin," which normally protects and insulates the nerve fibers of the spinal cord and brain, disappears in scattered patches during multiple sclerosis. Without this myelin, body signals go wrong. Hence the characteristics of multiple sclerosis may include shaking or tremor, extreme weakness, and progressive paralysis.

Mumps, infectious disease marked by swelling of the large salivary glands in front of the ears.

Signs of mumps appear between two and three weeks after exposure. The first sign is usually pain under one or both ears or under the chin. Often there is a fever, followed by swelling of one or more salivary glands— sometimes in the neck or throat, but usually just below and in front of the ears. Cases often start with chills, fever, headache, and loss of appetite for a day or two before the glands begin to swell. Most cases last about a week. A person with mumps is infectious from about a week before the glands start to swell until the swelling disappears.

Murmur, abnormal heart sound with a blowing or rasping quality.

Musca, fly.

Muscae Volitantes, spots before the eyes.

Muscle, the tissue that is responsible for body movement. The fibers forming the muscles are bound together in bundles of different lengths, breadths, and thicknesses. Bundles of muscle tissue can shorten, lengthen, or thicken. This type of action makes possible the movements of various parts of the body. There are two types of muscles. Voluntary muscles are those over which an individual can exert control, such as the muscles in the arms and legs. Involuntary muscles are those that an individual cannot control, such as the muscles of the heart and muscles involved in digestion and breathing. Muscles are attached to bones by strong, fibrous cords called tendons. Tendons are not elastic, but the power of contraction or extension of the muscles to which they are attached causes the bones forming joints to move either by flexing or by extending. The body has over six hundred muscles. Approximately forty percent of a male's weight is muscle. A female's weight is thirty-five percent muscle. The exact percentage depends on the physical condition of the individual. An athlete's weight will have a higher muscle percentage than that of an office worker.

Muscle Cramp, involuntary contraction of muscles.

Muscular, pertaining to muscle.

Muscular Dystrophy, a group of diseases, often called the muscular dystrophies, that cause a progressive wasting and weakening of the muscles. Muscular dystrophy weakens the voluntary muscles—the muscles on the outside of the body, such as the biceps of the arm. Unlike polio, the internal muscles, such as the diaphragm, are not affected by muscular dystrophy. Also, unlike polio, it usually affects equally the muscles on both sides of the body, leading to symmetrical weakening and wasting.
Muscular dystrophy has long been recognized as a disorder that often affects several people in one family. It is now well established that in most forms of muscular dystrophy an inherited characteristic coming from either parent is responsible.

Musculus, muscle.

Musophobia, extreme fear of mice.

Mussitation, delirious muttering.

Mustard Plaster, home remedy no longer commonly used.

Mutation, change.

Mute, unable to speak; one who cannot speak.

Mutism, speechlessness; dumbness.

Myalgia, muscle pain.

Myasthenia, muscle weakness.

Myatonia, muscle limpness.

Mycetismus, mushroom poisoning.

Mycology, science of fungi.

Mycosis, infection caused by fungi.

Mydriasis, abnormal pupil dilation.

Myectomy, surgical removal of a piece of muscle.

Myectopia, muscle displacement.

Myelauxe, bone marrow increase.

Myelin, the fatty covering that normally protects and insulates the nerve fibers of the spinal cord and brain. A breakdown of myelin is the cause of difficulty in multiple sclerosis. Without myelin, body signals to and from the nerves cannot function properly.

Myelon, spinal cord.

Myelopathy, disease of the spinal cord.

Myeloplegia, spinal paralysis.

Myelitis, spinal cord inflammation.

Myeloma, bone marrow tumor that may be cancerous.

Myenteron, muscular layer of the intestine.

Myiasia, condition when larvae of flies enter eyes, ears or intestines.

Myitis, muscle inflammation.

Myocardial Infarction, the damaging or death of a part of the heart muscle. Myocardial infarction is caused by a reduction or a complete stoppage of the blood supply to that area of the heart. Myocardial infarction is also known as heart attack, coronary occlusion, coronary, and coronary thrombosis. Acute myocardial infarction is the most frequent cardiac emergency. The incidence of myocardial infarction increases with advancing age, particularly after age fifty. The incidence is six times as high in males as in females.
In about half of the cases, onset is preceded by a history of angina pectoris. There is sudden severe pain in the chest, often radiating to the left arm. It usually persists for several hours. There is a fall in blood pressure and also shock. The pain is accompanied by pallor, sweating, and shortness of breath. Recovery from myocardial infarction generally requires absolute bed rest for four to six weeks. morphone or other drugs for the relief of pain and apprehension, and an anticoagulant medication. The total treatment time averages three to four months.

Myocarditis, inflammation of the heart muscle.

Myocardium, muscle that makes up the heart.

Myoclonus, muscle spasm.

Myocyte, cell of muscular tissue.

Myoid, resembling muscle.

Myology, study of muscles.

Myoma, tumor from muscle tissue.

Myomectomy, surgical removal of a myoma.

Myopathy, any muscle disease.

Myope, one who is nearsighted.

Myopia, nearsightedness. In the nearsighted eye, distant objects produce a blurred image. This is usually caused by an abnormally long front-to-back diameter of the eye. Thus, the focal image is formed in front of the retina.

Some cases of high myopia (where great correction is required) are progressive; they result from a disease rather than merely an error of refraction. Glasses may be unable to correct vision to normal range, and there may be destructive changes in various parts of the eye (choroid, retina, or vitreous body). High myopia tends to be accompanied by other changes that may be affected by strenuous physical activities.

Myosis, construction of the eye pupil.

Myositis, muscle inflammation, usually a voluntary muscle

Myospasm, muscle spasm.

Myotasis, stretching of muscle.

Myotonia, continuous muscle spasm not relieved by relaxation.

Myringitis, inflammation of the eardrum.

Myringotomy, incision into the eardrum.

Mythomania, habitual lying or exaggeration.

Myxedema, a form of cretinism occurring in adolescence or adulthood. The symptoms are similar—retardation, coarse hair, dry skin, and goiter. However, because it occurs after most growth has stopped, dwarfing is avoided. Like cretinism, myxedema is caused by a deficiency or a complete lack of thyroid hormone. Treatment consists of thyroid extract.

Myxoma, tumor of mucous tissue.

Myxorrhea, flow of mucus.

Myzesis, sucking.

Nail, a tough, dense modification of skin. Nails cover the ends of the fingers, thumbs, and toes. A nail grows out of its nail root. This root is embedded in the skin at the end of the nail closest to the body. The skin that covers the nail root and the sides of the nail is known as the nail wall. The tissue beneath the nail itself is referred to as the nail bed. The half-moon of white at the base of the nail is called the lunula. The rate of growth of nails is subject to individual differences. However, an individual's fingernails usually grow twice as fast as his toenails.

Nail Bed, part of a finger or toe covered by a nail.

Nail Biting, nervous tendency to bite or to chew the fingernails.

Naked, exposed to view.

Nalorphine, a drug classified as a narcotic antagonist.

Nanism, dwarfishness.

Nanus, dwarf; stunted.

Nap, short sleep.

Nape, back of the neck.

Narcissism, self love.

Narcolepsy, disease of unknown origin in which there are periodic episodes of sleep any time of day or night.

Narcomania, morbid desire for narcotics.

Narcosis, state of unconsciousness.

Narcotic, producing a state of unconsciousness; any sleep inducing drug; one addicted to the use of narcotics.

Narcotic Antagonists, a class of drugs that partially reverse the effects of narcotic drugs.
An overdose of a narcotic depresses the respiratory reflex. The narcotic antagonists are extremely effective in rapidly restoring the respiratory rate to its normal level. These drugs are also used in the detection of narcotic addiction. When a narcotic antagonist is given to a patient who is addicted to narcotics, the patient will exhibit the classical symptoms of withdrawal sickness.

Narcotize, to make unconscious.

Naris, nostril.

Nasal, pertaining to the nose; bone forming the bridge of the nose.

Nasal Cavity, the internal portion of the nose.

Nasus, nose.

Natal, pertaining to birth; pertaining to the buttocks.

Natality, birth rate.

Natant, floating.

Nathan's Test, a test for tuberculosis. A special serum, with a dressing, is applied to the surface of the arm. The dressing is removed the next day. A positive reaction will appear within six days.

Natis, buttocks.

Native, inherent; indigenous.

Natural, not artificial.

Natural Childbirth, a method of childbirth that requires the mother to be conscious and to cooperate actively with the processes of birth during labor and delivery. The expectant mother undergoes a program of education, exercise, and training (both physical and mental) in preparation for labor and delivery. The woman learns how to relax and to work in harmony with the contractions. Because natural childbirth requires little or no medication, there is little or no anesthesia in the mother's system for the baby to absorb.

Natural Immunity, the ability of a person to resist a disease without having had the disease and without being vaccinated against the disease. A natural immunity is based on the body's own defense and immunity system. The term is usually used to indicate an immunity to a disease that most people will contract when they are exposed to it.

Naturopathy, curing without drugs.

Nature Cure, any system of treatment which is based upon the belief that disease may best be cured and health maintained by the use of "natural remedies", as opposed to artificial and man-made drugs.

Naupathia, seasickness.

Nausea, stomach discomfort with the feeling of a need to vomit.

Nauseant, causing nausea.

Navel, remnant on outside of body where umbilical cord was attached at birth.

Near Point, point closest to the eye at which an object can be seen distinctly.

Nearsighted, able to see clearly only a short distance.

Nebula, haziness; cloudy urine.

Necator, hookworm.

Neck, part of the body connecting the head and trunk; narrow part near the extremity of any organ.
Located within the neck are body parts such as the pharynx, esophagus, larynx, trachea, and the thyroid gland. Thus, the neck is a continuation of both the digestive tract and the respiratory system. The organs mentioned above, as well as a number of lymph nodes, are situated in the front of the neck. The back of the neck consists of the spinal column. Within the spinal column are the spinal cord and a large number of nerves. Seven vertebrae form the beginning of the spinal column. These vertebrae, called the cervical vertebrae, are all located in the neck. The first cervical vertebra is referred to as the atlas. The construction of the atlas allows the head to tilt up and down, or nod. The second of the cervical vertebrae is known as the axis. This vertebra permits the head to turn from side to side. The rotation of the head pivots on the axis.
When the spinal cord is cut or subjected to extreme pressure, paralysis of the body occurs below the site of the injury. Therefore, any serious injury to the back of the neck can lead to paralysis from the neck down.

Necromania, obsession with death.

Necrophilism, intercourse with a corpse.

Necropneumonia, gangrene of lung.

Necropsy, autopsy.

Necrosis, death of a part of the body due to absence of blood supply.

Needle, pointed instrument for sewing or puncturing.

Negative Afterimage, the visual phenomenon that occurs after looking at a colored object and then at a white object. The afterimage will occur in the complimentary color.

Negativism, a symptom in mental diseases in which the patient resists or is against everything.

Neogala, first milk after childbirth.

Neogenesis, new formation.

Neonatal, concerning the newborn.

Neonatal Period, a term used to describe the first month of a baby's life.

Neonatorum, pertaining to the newborn.

Neonatus, a newborn infant.

Neopathy, new disease or complication.

Neophilism, excessive love of new things.

Neophobia, extreme fear of new things.

Neoplasm, an abnormal growth.

Nephralgia, pain in a kidney.

Nephrectomy, surgical removal of a kidney.

Nephrelcus, renal ulcer.

Nephric, pertaining to the kidney.

Nephritis, inflammation of the kidneys.

Nephrolithiases, formation of kidney stones.

Nephrology, study of the kidney.

Nephroma, tumor of the outer portion of the kidney.

Nephropexy, sewing a floating kidney into place.

Nephros, the kidney.

Nephrosis, disintegration of the kidney without signs of inflammation.

Nepiology, study of newborn.

Nerve, bundle of nerve fibers existing outside the central nervous system.

There are three different types of nerves. Each type fulfills a slightly different function. A sensory nerve receives sensations and transmits them to the brain. A motor nerve transmits impulses from the brain to the muscles and glands. An associative nerve transmits impulses from sensory nerves to motor nerves. The impulse moves from the dendrites, to the main cell body, to the axon. The impulse (which is actually a minute electrical charge) then jumps the space between the axon of one nerve cell and the dendrites of the next nerve cell. The small space between two nerves is called a synapse.

There are only eighty-six nerves in the entire body: twelve pairs of cranial nerves and thirty-one pairs of spinal nerves. All the remaining nerves in the body are only branches of the original eighty-six nerves.

Nerve Block, the anesthesia, or numbing, of an area of the body. This is accomplished by injecting the anesthesia in the vicinity of the region to be affected. Nerve blocks are performed for a variety of reasons, including the relief of pain in facial neuralgia and for prevention of pain when a dentist is filling or extracting a tooth.

Nervous, highly excitable.

Nervous, a condition of being easily disturbed or distressed.

Nervous System, the system that is responsible for keeping the various parts of the body and the organs controlling the body functions in touch with each other. The nervous system actually consists of two separate but interconnected and coordinated systems: the cerebrospinal system and the autonomic system. The cerebrospinal system consists of the brain and the spinal cord. The brain is a collection of nerve centers, each a central station for some part of the body — much like a central telephone station, with trunk lines or nerves connecting the parts of the body with their particular centers. Leaving the brain, these trunk nerves are bundled into the spinal cord, which passes down through the opening in the center of the backbone or spinal column, giving off branches to all parts and organs of the body. Most of the nerves entering and leaving the spinal cord are either sensory nerves or motor nerves. Sensory nerves enter the cord conveying impressions of sensations, such as heat, cold, touch, and pain, from different parts of the body to the brain. Motor nerves leave the spinal cord conveying impulses from the brain to the muscles causing movement. The autonomic system is a series of nerve centers in the chest and abdominal cavity along the spinal column. Each of these nerve centers, although interconnected with the cerebrospinal system, presides over and controls vital organs and vital functions. This system is not under control of the will, but through it involuntary muscles are stimulated to act alike during periods of wakefulness and during periods of sleep. Thus, the heart beats, respiration continues, blood pressure is maintained, food is digested, and the excretory organs function without any conscious effort. The autonomic nervous system consists of two sets of systems: the sympathetic nerves and the parasympathetic nerves. These two sets have opposite effects on the same body organs. For example, the parasympathetic nerves constrict the pupil of the eye; the sympathetic nerves dilate the pupil of the eye.

Nervus, pl., **Nervi,** nerve.

Network, structure composed of interlacing fibers.

Neural, pertaining to nerves or nervous tissue.

Neuralgia, a painful disorder of one or more nerves. The nerve causing the pain is not necessarily damaged. Neuralgia usually causes sharp, fitful pains. Facial neuralgia attacks persons over fifty years of age more frequently than it does younger people. In this disorder, excruciating pains flash intermittently across one side of the face. Sometimes a tingling of the skin warns that an attack is due. The spasms are usually "set off" by a draft of cold air or by swallowing, yawning, chewing, shaving, or similar activities. The pain can often be induced by pressing a sensitive "trigger point" along the nerve path. After a while, the painful flashes stop, only to appear again at any time from hours to months later. If the condition is not relieved, the period between attacks becomes shorter and shorter, until pain is practically continuous. Various infections or injuries of the nerve may cause neuralgia to strike other parts of the body. Sometimes the back of the neck, the eye, the lower back, or the chest may be involved. The symptoms may suggest other diseases. Sharp chest pains, for example, may suggest heart disease or pleurisy when they are actually caused by neuralgia. An experienced physician can identify true neuralgia.

Neurasthenia, exhaustion of the nerves.

Neure, neuron.

Neurectasia, stretching of a nerve to relieve pain.

Neuritis, a disorder of one or more nerves. Neuritis usually involves inflammation of a nerve or nerves and causes a constant, burning pain.
  The disorder may be localized to one nerve or may involve many. Either type may result from injuries, poisons, infections, or chilling. The localized type is more common. The path of the nerve develops a burning sensation. The flesh may have a numb or "crawling" feeling. The skin is often reddened along the course of the nerve. The condition is not usually serious unless it is allowed to continue without treatment. Sciatica is a localized neuritis of the sciatic nerve. This is the nerve that runs along the back of the leg. A generalized neuritis is far more serious than a localized neuritis. It is often caused by prolonged illness, by exposure to chemicals such as lead or arsenic, or by alcoholism. Failure to eat and absorb enough food containing the B vitamins seems to be an important cause. Usually the patient complains for several weeks of

numbness, tingling in the fingers and feet, and of sensations of heat and cold. There may be a slight fever. After the initial symptoms, the patient experiences weakness and pain in the muscles. If untreated, he may lose all feeling in the "glove and stocking" areas of the arms and legs and develop paralysis. The untreated patient may eventually become bedridden. Neuritis may occasionally be relieved by an operation to remove the cause (such as a tumor). A sound, carefully planned exercise program is often prescribed in addition to a variety of drugs.

Neuroblastoma, a malignant tumor of the nervous system; it is composed of immature nerve cells.

Neurocirculatory Asthenia, a complex of nervous and circulatory symptoms, often involving a sense of fatigue, dizziness, shortness of breath, rapid heartbeat, and nervousness. Neurocirculatory asthenia is also known as effort syndrome and soldier's heart.

Neurocranium, portion of the cranium enclosing the brain.

Neurocyte, any nerve cell.

Neurodynamic, pertaining to nervous energy.

Neurogenic, a term used to indicate anything that originates from within the nervous system.

Neuroid, resembling a nerve.

Neuro-induction, mental suggestion.

Neurologist, specialist in disorders of the nervous system.

Neuroma, tumor composed of nerve substance.

Neuromuscular, pertaining to the nerves and muscles.

Neuron, nerve cell.

Neuronitis, inflammation of a neuron.

Neuropathy, any disease of the nervous system.

Neurophthisis, degeneration or wasting of nerve tissue.

Neuroplasm, protoplasm of a nerve cell.

Neuropsychiatry, branch of medicine dealing with nervous and mental disorders.

Neurosis, minor mental disorder.

Neurospasm, muscular twitching.

Neurosurgeon, specialist in surgery of the brain and nervous system.

Neurosyphilis, syphilis of the nervous system.

Neurothlipsis, nerve pressure.

Neurotrauma, nerve lesion.

Nevus, relatively small benign growths on the skin. They are commonly referred to as moles, birthmarks, freckles, etc., depending on the consistency, color of pigmentation, and degree of elevation. Some nevi have a tendency to become malignant. These are usually flat, dark moles that do not have hairs. Additionally, they are usually located in areas that receive constant friction from clothes, other skin, or foreign objects. Areas of special concern are the palms of the hands and the soles of the feet.

Nexus, a binding together.

Niche, depression; recess.

Nicotine, poisonous alkaloid of tobacco.
Nicotine affects the autonomic nervous system. It affects both the parasympathetic and the sympathetic nerves. Thus, the pupils of the eyes are first constricted and then dilated.

Nictitation, excessive winking.

Nidus, cluster, focus of infection; nerve nucleus.

Niemann-Pick Disease, a form of mental illness characterized by a defect of metabolism of fats. This disease is inherited. The symptoms include a brownish discoloration of the skin and progressive blindness. Niemann-Pick disease, sometimes known as lipoid histiocytosis, often causes early death.

Night Cry, cry of a child during sleep.

Nightmare, bad dream.

Nightwalking, sleepwalking.

Nigra, black.

Nigrities Linguae, black tongue.

N.I.H., National Institutes of Health.

Niphablepsia, snow blindness.

Nipple, protuberance in each breast from which the female secretes milk.

Nit, egg of a louse.

Nitrites, a group of chemical compounds, many of which cause dilation of the small blood vessels.
The importance of these compounds is that by dilating the blood vessels, they reduce the resistance to the flow of blood and consequently lower the blood pressure.

Nitroglycerin, a drug (one of the nitrites) that relaxes the muscles in the blood vessels. Nitroglycerin is used to relieve attacks of angina pectoris and spasm of the coronary arteries. Nitroglycerin works by relaxing and dilating blood vessels. This allows blood to flow more easily through the vessels, and consequently lowers the blood pressure and reduces the work load of the heart muscle. Nitroglycerin is probably the best and most widely used drug for the relief of pain in angina attacks. It is taken in tablet form, either under the tongue (where it quickly dissolves) or chewed. Nitroglycerin will not do its job if it is simply swallowed in tablet form. Most patients experience total cessation of pain within two minutes.

N.L.N., National League for Nursing.

Noctophobia, extreme fear of night.

Nocturia, bed wetting; frequent urination at night.

Nocturnal Emission, the involuntary ejaculation of semen during sleep.

Nocuity, harmfulness.

Node, small rounded protuberance; point of constriction.

Nodule, small node; small group of cells.

Nodus, node.

Noma, form of gangrene of the mouth found in ill-nourished or weak children.

Non Compos Mentis, not of sound mind.

Non Repetat, do not repeat.

Nonsexual, without sex, asexual.

Nontoxic, not poisonous.

Nonunion, failure of bone fragments to knit together.

Nonviable, incapable.

Noopsyche, intellectual processes.

Norepinephrine, a hormone secreted by the adrenal glands. Norepinephrine produces a rise in blood pressure by constricting the small blood vessels.

Norm, standard.

Normal, a term used to indicate something that falls within a regular or established pattern. The concept of normalcy is a very difficult one in medicine. What is normal for one person is not necessarily normal for another person. Physicians refer to certain reactions to certain drugs as normal reactions. This means that most people have these reactions. For example, most people experience a certain amount of pain relief from aspirin. That is the normal reaction. However, some people are allergic to aspirin and their response to it may include an upset stomach or a rash, as well as more violent reactions. When compared with the average reaction, theirs is not normal, but their body is reacting normally for them. Another example is the range of individual differences in body temperature. Normal, or average, body temperature is 98.6°F. when taken orally. Anything below that is called subnormal; anything above that is referred to as a fever. However, there are people whose temperature is normally (for them) 98°F. or even lower. They are perfectly healthy, but their temperature is not normal. When people like this report a temperature of 98.6°F., they are usually running a fever, even though their temperature is normal for most people. An experienced physician is always aware of individual differences. He uses the concept of normal as a yardstick to compare an individual's reactions, not as a rule to which all patients must adhere. One of the reasons medicine is considered to be an art as well as a science is the degree to which these individual differences affect diagnosis and treatment.

Normocyte, normal sized red blood cell.

Normoptopic, normally located.

Normotensive, any condition characterized by normal blood pressure.

Nose, organ of the sense of smell.

Nosebleed, hemorrhage from the nose.

Nose Drops, medicine taken in liquid form through the nose. Nose drops are usually used to help clear the sinus passages and allow free breathing.

Nosema, sickness; disease.

Nosology, science of disease classification.

Nosophilia, extreme desire to be sick.

Nosophobia, extreme fear of illness.

Nosopoietic, causing disease.

Nostalgia, homesickness; feeling for past experiences and things.

Nostomania, extreme homesickness.

Nostril, nasal aperture.

Nostrum, patent medicine.

Notal, dorsal.

Notalgia, back pain.

Notifiable, pertaining to any disease which must be reported to health authorities.

Notochord, the first supportive structure of an embryo.

Noxious, harmful; deadly; poisonous.

Nubile, of childbearing age.

Nucha, nape of the neck.

Nucleus, pl., **Neuclei,** center of a cell.

Nudomania, extreme desire to be nude.

Nudophobia, extreme fear of being nude.

Nullipara, woman who has not given birth to a child.

Numb, insensible.

Numbness, a condition in which an area of the body is insensitive when touched. Numbness can be caused by disease, malfunctioning body parts, etc. Numbness can also be artificially induced by drugs to relieve existing pain or to prevent pain during a surgical or dental procedure. The sensation of touch and external pressure is transmitted by nerves. When the nerves are damaged or blocked (as by an anesthetic), the brain does not receive the proper information from the affected nerves. The term numbness is usually used to indicate a loss of surface and subsurface feeling. This can be very dangerous, because part of the body's warning system is lost. Thus, if a patient with a numb finger is burned, he may not realize it until the deep nerves are affected. By the time the deep nerves are alerted, very serious damage may have been sustained.

Nurse, one who is trained to care for the sick; to care for the sick; to breast feed.

Nutation, nodding.

Nutrient, nourishing.

Nutrition, the combination of processes by which a living organism receives and utilizes the materials necessary for the maintenance of its functions and for the growth and renewal of its components. From simple one-celled plants to highly complex human beings, all living things need food. Food is necessary to support growth, to repair constantly wearing tissues, and to supply energy for physical activity. Unless the food consumed supplies all the elements required for normal life processes, the human body cannot operate at peak efficiency for very long. If an essential nutrient is missing from the diet over long periods of time, deficiency diseases such as rickets, scurvy, or certain anemias may develop. Everyone needs the same nutrients throughout life but in different amounts. Proportionately greater amounts are required for the growth of a body than just for its upkeep. Boys and men need more energy and nutrients than girls and women. Large people need more than small people. Active people require more food energy than inactive ones. People recovering from illness need more than healthy people. The nutrients in food that are necessary for good health can be divided into certain groups — proteins, carbohydrates, fats, vitamins, minerals, and water. Most common foods consist of combinations of the above. Foods that are good sources of one food element usually also contribute other essential elements as well, but no one food supplies all needed nutrients in sufficient amounts. For good nutrition all essential food elements must work together. Therefore, well-balanced nutrition calls for a well-chosen variety of foods. Good nutrition is just as important for older people as it is for infants and growing teenagers. However, some of the nutritional requirements do change in elderly people. Usually, less physical work is performed in advanced age, and therefore the body's requirements for calories is lower. Dietary calories that are not used are stored in the form of body fat, and many persons who continue the richer diet of their physically more active days may become too heavy. This is the main reason why fewer carbohydrates and less fat are needed in the food of the aged.

Nutritious, giving nourishment.

Nux, nut.

Nyctalgia, pain during the night.

Nyctalopia, the inability to see at night or in a low-light level. Nyctalopia is also known as night blindness. The ability of the eye to see at night or in a dark room depends on the rods in the retina. The rods transmit black, white, and gray impulses. When the rods are not functioning properly, there is no low-light vision (color- and bright-light vision are not affected by the rods). Nyctalopia is caused by a lack of rhodopsin, a substance formed from vitamin A. Night blindness can also be an inherited condition.

Nycterine, occurring at night.

Nyctophobia, extreme fear of darkness.

Nyctotyphlosis, night blindness.

Nygma, puncture wound.

Nymphectomy, surgical removal of the small lips of the vagina.

Nymphomania, excessive sexual desire in the female.

Nystagmus, jerking movement of the eyes which may be inborn or a sign of disease of the nervous system.

Nyxis, puncture; pricking.

Oaric, concerning the ovary.

Oaritis, ovarian inflammation.

Obdormition, numbness and tingling in an arm or leg.

Obduction, autopsy.

Obesity, a bodily condition in which there is an excess of fat in relation to other body components. The condition is presumed to exist when an individual is twenty percent or more over normal weight. Obesity is caused by a persistent caloric intake that exceeds the energy output needs of the body. Causation is a complex problem, but current knowledge includes such factors as heredity, emotions, culture, diet, and lack of exercise.
Reduced to simple terms, the successful treatment of obesity involves achieving a balance between diet and exercise.

Obfuscation, confusion.

Oblique, diagonal.

Obliteration, complete surgical removal of a part; total memory loss.

Obmutescence, loss of power to speak.

Obnubilation, confused state.

Obsession, all consuming emotion or idea.

Obstetrical, pertaining to obstetrics.

Obstetrician, physician who specializes in pregnant women.

Obstetrics, branch of medicine dealing with pregnancy and delivery of infants.

Obstipation, constipation due to obstruction.

Obstruction, a term indicating the blockage of a body vessel. Obstructions can occur in any body vessel. They can be very serious, and, if they occur in certain places, they can be fatal. For example, a child who swallows something solid may find his trachea obstructed or blocked. Unless the object is removed or an alternate breathing passage is made (tracheostomy), the child may die from lack of air. A blood clot formed in another part of the body may be carried to one of the arteries of the brain, where it obstructs the further flow of blood and causes a stroke. Obstructions may be caused by foreign objects, by blood clots, by naturally formed "stones" (such as gallstones), and by tumors (benign or malignant).

Obtund, to dull sensation.

Obturation, closing of an opening.

Occipital, pertaining to the bone that constitutes the back part of the skull.

Occiput, back part of skull.

Occlude, to block or obstruct.

Occlusion, shutting; the full meeting of the chewing surfaces of the upper and lower teeth.

Occult, hidden; obscure.

Occupational Disease, disease caused by one's work.

Occupational Therapy, use of an activity as treatment.

Ochlesis, disease due to overcrowding.

Ochlophobia, extreme fear of crowds.

Ochrodermia, yellowness of the skin.

Octoroon, one who is ⅛ Negro and ⅞ Caucasian.

Ocular, pertaining to the eye or vision.

Oculist, specialist in eye diseases.

Oculus, eye.

Odaxesmus, biting of tongue or skin of mouth during a fit.

Odaxitic, stinging or itching.

Odonitis, tooth inflanmation.

Odontalgia, toothache.

Odontechtomy, tooth extraction.

Odonterism, chattering of teeth.

Odontexesis, cleaning of teeth.

Odontiasis, teething.

Odontic, pertaining to the teeth.

Odontoclasis, breaking a tooth.

Odontodynia, toothache.

Odontogeny, development of teeth.

Odontology, study of the teeth.

Odontoma, tumor arising from the same tissue from which teeth are formed.

Odontoprisis, grinding teeth.

Odontotomy, incision of a tooth.

Odontotrypy, drilling of a tooth.

Odynophagia, pain with swallowing.

Odynophobia, extreme fear of pain.

Oedipus Complex, abnormal love of a child for a parent of the opposite sex, usually a boy for his mother.

Oikophobia, extreme hatred of the home.

Ointment, soft fat substance spread on skin as therapy.

Oleaginous, oily.

Olecranon, bony inner portion of elbow.

Oleum, oil.

Olfaction, smelling; sense of smell.

Olfactory, pertaining to the sense of smell.

Olfactory Nerve, the cranial nerve that transmits the sense of smell from the nose to the brain.

Oligemia, deficiency of blood.

Oligocholia, bile deficiency.

Oligogalactia, deficient milk secretion.

Oligoposy, insufficient liquid intake.

Oligotrichia, lack of hair.

Oligotrophy, insufficient nutrition.

Oliguria, decreased amount of urine production.

Omagra, shoulder gout.

Omalgia, neuralgia of the shoulder.

Omentum, large fatty membrane which acts as a cover for the bowels.

Omitis, shoulder, inflammation.

Omnivorous, eating all types of food.

Omodynia, shoulder pain.

Omphalic, pertaining to the umbilicus.

Omphalitis, inflammation of the navel.

Omphalocele, hernia around navel.

Omphalos, navel.

Onanism, complete sexual intercourse with ejaculation outside the vagina; masturbation.

Oncology, the branch of medicine that is concerned with tumors.

Oncosis, multiple tumors.

Oncocyte, tumor cell.

Oncogenous, causing tumors.

Oncoma, tumor.

Oncosis, multiple tumors.

Oncotic, pertaining to swelling.

Oneiric, pertaining to dreams.

Oniomania, excessive desire to buy things.

Onomatomania, compulsion to repeat words.

Onychia, infection and inflammation around fingernails.

Onychophagia, nail biting.

Onychosis, disease of the nails.

Onyx, fingernail; toenail.

Onyxis, ingrown nails.

Oocyesis, pregnancy in the ovary.

Oophoralgia, ovarian pain.

Oophorectomy, surgical removal of an ovary.

Oophoritis, inflammation of an ovary.

Oophoroma, malignant ovarian tumor.

Oophoron, ovary.

Oosperm, fertilized ovum.

Ootheca, ovary.

Opaque, dark; not transparent; mentally dull.

Open-Heart Surgery, surgery performed on the open heart while the bloodstream is diverted through a heart-lung machine.

Open Wound, any break in the skin. When the skin is un-broken, it affords protection from most infections, bacteria, or germs. However, when the skin is broken, no matter how slight the break, germs may enter, and an infection may develop. Any wound where the skin is broken should receive prompt medical attention, and only sterile objects should be in contact with any open wounds. If germ life has been carried into an open wound by the object causing the break in the skin, nature attempts to wash out the germs by the flow of blood; but some types of wounds do not bleed freely. A break in the skin may range from a pin puncture or scratch to an extensive cut, tear, or mash. An open wound may be only the surface evidence of a more serious injury to deeper structures, such as fractures, particularly in head injuries involving fracture of the skull. In first aid, open wounds are divided into four classifications: abrasions, incised wounds, lacerated wounds, and punctured wounds.

Operable, capable of being relieved by an operation.

Operation, surgical procedure.

Operation Major, one in which there is considerable risk to life.

Operation, Minor, one in which there is little or no danger to life.

Ophidism, snake poisoning.

Ophthalic, pertaining to the eyes.

Ophthalmia, inflammation of the eye.

Ophthalmologist, specialist in the eye and its diseases.

Ophthalmology, study of eye and its diseases.

Ophthalmoplegia, paralysis of the eye muscles.

Ophthalmoscope, instrument for examining the eyes.

Opiate, any opium derivative.

Opisthotonis, arched-back position with head and heel on the horizontal.

Opium, the powder produced by drying the seeds of *Papaver somniferum,* the poppy plant that grows in the Near East. Raw opium has been used as a pain-killer for thousands of years. It has also been used in the treatment of dysentery. However, not until the early part of the nineteenth century were the potent derivatives of opium isolated: morphine in 1803, codeine in 1832, and papaverine in 1848.
Opium and its derivatives are narcotics or pain-reducers. They are physically and sometimes psychologically addictive. Despite the dangers inherent in their use, the opium derivatives are the most effective narcotic agents known to man.

Opsialgia, pain in region of face.

Opsomania, extreme craving for a particular food.

Optic, concerning sight or eye.

Optical, pertaining to vision.

Optician, one who makes lenses or optical instruments.

Optic Nerve, the nerve that transmits sight impulses from the retina of the eye to the brain.

O.R., operating room.

Ora, border; margin.

Orad, toward the mouth.

Oral, pertaining to the mouth.

Oral Contraception (the "pill"), one of the most effective methods of birth control. Each pill contains hormones which causes the ovaries to stop releasing eggs.

Orbicular, circular.

Orbit, eyesocket.

Orchiectomy, surgical removal of a testes.

Orchiodynia, testicle pain.

Orchioncus, tumor of a testes.

Orchis, testicle.

Orchitis, inflammation of the testicle.

Orderly, a male hospital attendant.

Orexigenic, appetite stimulant.

Organ, group of tissue with specific function.

Organic Heart Disease, a heart disease that is caused by some structural abnormality in the heart or circulatory system.

Organism, individual animal or plant.

Orgasm, sexual climax.

Orifice, opening, entrance.

Oropharynx, first part of throat starting at mouth.

Orotherapy, treatment with serums.

Orrhorrhea, watery discharge; flow of serum.

Orrhology, study of blood serum.

Orthodontics, the branch of dentistry that deals with uneven bites or malocclusion.

Orthogenics, eugenics.

Orthopedics, branch of medicine dealing with the surgery of bones and joints.

Orthopedist, specialist in orthopedics.

Orthosis, correction of a deformity.

Orthostatic, concerning standing position.

Orthopnea, condition in which difficult breathing is aided by propping up head and shoulders.

Orthopsychiatry, branch of psychiatry dealing mainly with adolescents.

Orthuria, normal frequency of urination.

Os, pl., Ora, mouth opening.

Os, pl., **Ossa,** bone.

Oscedo, yawning; white spots in the mouth.

Oscheitis, inflammation of the scrotum.

Oscillometer, an instrument that measures the changes in magnitude of the pulsations in the arteries.

Oscitation, yawning.

Osculation, kissing; joining of two structures by their mouths.

Osculum, aperature.

Osmatic, having an acute sense of smell.

Osmesis, smelling.

Osmics, science of odors.

Osmosis, the diffusion (or movement) of a fluid through a membrane from an area of higher pressure to an area of lower pressure. The membranes through which osmosis can take place are called semipermeable membranes. These semipermeable membranes allow fluids and small molecules to pass through them, but they block the passage of larger molecules. Thus, these membranes act as a sieve. In the human body, cell membranes are semipermeable and permit this diffusion. Oxygen, blood, and digested nutrients pass through cells by osmosis, providing energy for growth and replacement as well as for regular life processes. Blood is pumped under pressure from the heart to the large arteries. From the arteries, blood passes into even smaller blood vessels, called capillaries. By the time blood reaches the capillaries, the pressure has been considerably reduced. However, the pressure of the blood in the capillaries is still greater than the fluid in the cells. Hence, through the process of osmosis, blood in the capillaries enters the individual cells. The movement of fluids, waste material, etc. through the body tissues is a result of osmosis. Waste materials are removed from the blood in the kidneys through this same process.

Osphresis, sense of smell.

Osphus, loin.

Ossa, bones.

Osseous, bonelike.

Ossicle, small bone of ear.

Ossiferous, producing bone.

Ossification, bone formation; change of tissue to bone.

Ossify, to turn into bone.

Ostectomy, surgical removal of a bone.

Osteitis, bone inflammation.

Osteoarthritis, a degenerative joint disease. Osteoarthritis seems to be caused by a combination of aging, irritation of the joints, and normal wear and tear. It is far commoner than rheumatoid arthritis, but, as a rule, it is less damaging. Older people are more likely to have osteoarthritis than are younger people. Chronic irritation of the joints is the main contributing factor. This may result from overweight, poor posture, injury, or strain from one's occupation or recreation.

The primary characteristic of osteoarthritis is degeneration of joint cartilage. This becomes soft and wears unevenly. In some areas it may wear away completely, exposing the underlying bone. Thickening of the ends of the bones may also occur. The remainder of the body is seldom affected. Except in some cases that involve the hip joints or knees, the disease seldom causes serious deformity or crippling.

Common symptoms are pain, aches, and stiffness. Pain is usually experienced when certain joints are used, especially finger joints and those that bear the body's weight. Enlargement of the fingers at the last joint often occurs. Although permanent, enlargements (nodes) of this type seldom lead to disability.

Osteocarcinoma, bone cancer.

Osteochrondritis, inflammation of both bone and cartilage from which bone is formed.

Osteochrondroma, tumor arising from bone cartilage.

Osteology, study of bones.

Osteoma, tumor composed of various parts of bone.

Osteomalacia, softening of bone.

Osteomyelitis, an inflammatory disease of bone caused usually by infection with streptococcus or staphylococcus.

Osteomyelitis can occur after a bone has been fractured and one of the broken ends of the bone pierces the skin. The open end of the bone may then be exposed to microorganisms capable of causing this infection. Before the discovery of antibiotics, osteomyelitis was often caused by a serious infection in another part of the body that spread to the bone or bones. Today, most infections are cured before they can enter the bloodstream and attack the bones. The symptoms of osteomyelitis are sudden pain in the bone and an elevated temperature. Treatment consists of chemotherapy—usually penicillin when the diagnosis is made before the infection spreads too far into the bone marrow. If the infection has spread, drainage of the affected bone may be needed in addition to the drugs. When the infection is severe, parts of the bone may have to be removed.

Osteopathy, system of treatment based on the idea that diseases are caused by minor dislocations of the spine, and, therefore, curable by bone manipulation.

Osteoporosis, a disorder that causes a gradual decrease in both the amount and strength of bone tissue. The bones usually involved first in osteoporosis are those of the spine and pelvis. Ordinarily, the disease thins individual bones of the spine, which are then compressed by the weight of the body and eventually reach the point of outright fracture and collapse. At any stage of osteoporosis the patient may have chronic low-back pain. As the disease advances, the patient's back becomes deformed, the patient grows progressively shorter, and capacity for physical activity becomes more and more limited. Also as the disease progresses, other bones become thinned, particularly those of the legs and arms. Because the affected bones are weak and porous, often breaking under even minor stress, the disease is responsible for many of the fractures experienced by elderly people. Osteoporosis is often the real cause of the numerous broken hips that hospitalize so many older people for long periods and which, in many cases, begin their physical decline. This disease is one of the major causes of physical disability in old age.

Osteosis, formation of bony tissue.

Ostium, small opening.

Ostum, vaginal, outer opening of the vagina.

O.T., occupational therapy.

Otalgia, earache.

Otic, pertaining to the ear.

Otitis, inflammation of the ear.

Otitis Media, an infection of the middle ear, frequently caused by the spread of bacterial infection from the throat.

Otolaryngology, medical specialty concerned with ear, nose and throat.

Otologist, ear specialist.

Otology, branch of medicine dealing with the ear.

Otopathy, any ear disease.

Otosclerosis, type of deafness caused by hardening of the tissues and bones in the inner ear.

Otoscope, instrument used to examine ear.

Oula, the gums.

Ouloid, scar-like.

Outer Ear, the part of the ear that includes the external ear and the external auditory canal.

Outlay, graft.

Outpatient, one who received treatment at a hospital without being admitted.

Oval, egg-shaped.

Oval Window, an opening in the wall of the bone housing the inner ear.

Ovarian, pertaining to the ovaries.

Ovariectomy, surgical removal of an ovary.

Ovary, the two small female organs that produce ova, the female sex cells or eggs. An ovary is about the size and shape of an almond. The ovaries are located at the outer end of the fallopian tubes—one to the right and one to the left.
Each ovary contains about 300,000 ova. Out of this large supply, only about 400 actually reach maturity during a woman's life. Of these 400, only a few are finally fertilized and go on to become human beings. About every twenty-eight days, midway between two menstrual cycles (about fourteen days before the menstrual flow), a single ovum leaves one of the ovaries. The two ovaries alternate: one month the ovum is released from the right ovary; the next month an ovum is released from the left ovary. This cycle repeats itself, except during pregnancies, until the menopause, when the childbearing part of a woman's life comes to an end.

Ovate, oval.

Overdose, taking more of a drug or drugs than the body can safely handle.

Overgrowth, excessive growth.

Overweight, exceeding desired weight by more than 10%.

Oviduct, tube from ovary to uterus.

Ovulation, process of discharge of egg from ovary.

Ovum, pl., **Ova,** egg cell.

Oxyblepsia, very acute vision.

Oxycinesia, pain on motion.

Oxygen, an element needed for life which is brought into the body by the process of breathing.

Oxygeusia, acute sense of taste.

Oxylalia, rapid speech.

Oxyopia, acute sight.

Oxytocic, agent used to stimulate uterus to contract.

Ozostomia, offensive breath.

Ozena, disease of nasal passage leading to the production of a foul-smelling discharge.

Ozone, a form of oxygen. Under ordinary conditions it is a colorless or pale-blue gas and has a characteristic pungent odor. In high concentrations it is extremely flammable, and in liquid form it becomes a dangerous explosive. As a strong oxidizing agent, ozone has many uses. Its greatest use is in the suppression of mold and bacterial growth, such as in the treatment of drinking-water supplies and industrial wastes, and the sterilizing of food products. Other uses of ozone include the rapid aging of wood; the aging of liquor; rapid drying of varnishes and printing ink; production of peroxides; bleaching of oils, waxes, textiles, and papers; and deodorizing of feathers. Despite its usefulness, ozone is acutely and chronically toxic to humans. Workers in enclosed spaces where ozone is produced or used should be on guard against the potential hazards to which they may be accidentally exposed.

Pabulum, food, nourishment.

Pacemaker, a small mass of specialized cells in the right upper chamber of the heart. These cells are responsible for the electrical impulses that initiate the contractions of the heart. The natural pacemaker is also called the sinoatrial node or the S-A node of Keith-Flack. The term pacemaker, or, more exactly, electric cardiac pacemaker, or electric pacemaker, is also applied to an electrical device that can be substituted for a defective natural pacemaker. The artificial pacemaker controls the beat of the heart by a series of rhythmic electrical discharges that replace the missing natural electrical impulses. If the electrodes that deliver the discharges to the heart are placed on the outside of the chest, the device is called an external pacemaker. If the electrodes are placed within the chest wall, it is called an internal pacemaker. An internal pacemaker is surgically implanted in the chest. It is a self-contained unit, requiring only periodic battery changes.

Pachyblepharon, thickening of the eyelid.

Pachycephalous, thick wall.

Pachychilla, thick lips.

Pachyderma, thick skin.

Pachyglossia, thick tongue.

Pachyhemia, thickening of the blood.

Pachymeningitis, inflammation of the outer covering of the brain and spinal cord.

Pachymeter, instrument for measuring thickness.

Pachynsis, thickening.

Pachyonychia, thickening of the nails.

Pachypodous, big feet.

Pack, a dry or wet, hot or cold blanket wrapped around the patient.

Packing, material used to fill wound or cavity.

Pad, soft cushion.

Paget's Disease; Osteitis Deformans, thickening of bones, mainly skull and shin; rash of nipple connected with breast tumor.

Pain, an elementary sensation of physical suffering. The sensation of pain is part of the protective system of the body. Pain serves as a warning of bodily damage, disease, or malfunction. When the body experiences pain and there is no apparent external cause, the pain itself is a warning to consult a physician. Frequently, there is no visible manifestation of the source of the pain—such as a burn or a wound. The lack of physical evidence indicates the possibility of disease or malfunction. Pain or the sensation of pain occurs in the brain. Consequently, if there is no brain, or if the brain is depressed by drugs (as by a general anesthetic) or by injury, there is no sensation of pain. Naturally, once the brain returns to normal, the sensation of pain returns. At the same time, if the nerves do not send a warning to the brain, the brain cannot initiate the pain sensation. Some pain has no physical (internal or external) basis. This pain is said to be psychogenic or psychosomatic. This type of pain—as intense as if it were caused by a physical stimulus—is caused by emotional disorders. Another type of pain, known as neurogenic, can be very confusing, because, like psychogenic pain, it mimics pain from a physical stimulus. Unlike psychosomatic pain, neurogenic pain has a physical basis, although not necessarily in the painful area. Neurogenic pain results from an improper functioning of one or more of the nerves.

Pain, False, false labor pains.

Palantine, pertaining to the palate.

Palate, roof of the mouth divided into hard and soft portions.

Palatitis, inflammation of the palate.

Paleontology, study of early man.

Palliate, to reduce or allay discomfort.

Palliative, relieving pain or suffering.

Pallid, lacking.

Pallor, paleness of skin.

Palm, inside portion of hand.

Palma, palm.

Palmar, pertaining to the palm.

Palpable, able to be touched.

Palpate, to examine by feeling.

Palpebra, eyelid.

Palpebra Inferior, lower eyelid.

Palpebra Superior, upper eyelid.

Palpitation, rapid pulsation in an organ, usually refers to the heart.

Palsy, impaired function or paralysis.

Paludism, malaria.

Panacea, cure for all ills.

Panarthritis, inflammation of the entire joint.

Pancarditis, infection of all parts of heart.

Panchrest, panacea.

Pancreas, gland lying behind and below the stomach which produces ferments which are passed into the intestinal tract to help in digestion; site of insulin production.

Pancreatitis, inflammation of the pancreas.

Pancreectomy, removal of pancreas in part or whole.

Pandemic, the spread of an infectious disease over a wide area. A pandemic is larger than an epidemic. The term is usually restricted to diseases that spread over all or almost all the world. Outbreaks of influenza have been pandemic.

Pandiculation, stretching and yawning.

Panesthesia, all of the sensations experienced.

Pang, spontaneous, sudden emotion or pain.

Panhidrosis, perspiration over entire body.

Panhysterectomy, complete removal of the womb.

Panic, extreme anxiety, with temporary loss of reason.

Panniculitis, inflammation of abdominal wall fat.

Panniculus, layer of tissue, fatty layer.

Pannus, abnormal membrane on the cornea.

Panophobia, extreme fear of everything in general.

Pansinusitis, inflammation of all the sinuses.

Pant, breathe fast and hard.

Pap, nipple; soft food.

Papaverine, a drug derived from opium. Papaverine is a muscle relaxant.

Papilla, nipple-like protuberance.

Papilla, Mammary, breast nipple.

Papillary Muscles, small bundles of muscles in the wall of the lower chambers of the heart to which the cords leading to the cusps of the valves (chordae tendineae) are attached.

Papilledema, swelling of optic nerve where nerve enters eye.

Papilloma, benign tumor of skin or inner membranes.

Pap Smear, a technique developed chiefly by Dr. George N. Papanicolaou (1883-1962) that involves the microscopic examination of cells collected from the vagina. The Pap smear is an excellent technique for the early detection of cancer of the uterine cervix, or neck of the womb. In fact, the Pap smear is one of the major reasons for the decrease in deaths from cancer of the uterine cervix. Gynecologists now routinely do a Pap smear as part of the annual examination of female patients.

Papule, small red raised area on skin.   .

Par, pair.

Para- (prefix), beside.

Paracentesis, puncture.

Parachroma, skin discoloration.

Paracusia, any hearing defect.

Paracyesis, pregnancy outside uterus.

Paralalia, speech disorder.

Paraldehyde, a drug that acts as a sedative and hypnotic.

Paralgesia, painful sensation.

Paralysis, loss of the power of movement or sensation in one or more parts of the body.

Paralytic, pertaining to paralysis.

Paralyze, to cause loss of muscle control and/or feeling.

Paramenia, irregular or abnormal menstrual period.

Parametrium, tissue surrounding and supporting the womb.

Paranoia, chronic psychosis characterized by fears, suspicion and well organized imaginery thoughts.

Paraphemia, distorted speech.

Paraphobia, mild phobia.

Paraplegia, the loss of both motion and sensation in the legs and lower part of the body. This condition is the result of a disease or injury to the spinal column. Among the diseases capable of causing paraplegia are poliomyelitis, muscular dystrophy, multiple sclerosis, and tumors of the spinal cord. Principal traumatic (or accidental) causes include birth injuries, automobile accidents, airplane crashes, gunshot or shrapnel wounds, and falls or injuries in industry and sports. The loss of motion and sensation occurs from the site of the disease or damage to the spinal cord downward. Additionally, there may be a loss of normal control of the bowels and bladder.

Parapoplexy, slight apoplexy.

Parasite, any animal or plant which lives inside or on the body of another animal or plant.

Parasympathetic Nervous System, a subdivision of the autonomic or involuntary nervous system.

Parateresiomania, compulsion to see new sights.

Parathymia, disordered emotion.

Parathyroid Glands, group of six small glands situated around the thyroid gland concerned with calcium and phosphorus in body.
Diminished function or removal of the parathyroid glands results in a low calcium level in the blood. In extreme cases death occurs; it is preceded by strong contractions of the muscles and by convulsions.

Paregoric, derivative of opium used to help relieve pain or diarrhea.

Parenchyma, productive part of an organ.

Parent, one who begets offspring.

Parenteral, outside of digestive tract.

Paresis, paralysis due to disease of brain, usually syphilis.

Paries, wall of a cavity.

Parietal Pericardium, a thin membrane sac that surrounds the heart and roots of the great vessels.

Pareunia, sexual intercourse.

Parity, capable of bearing children.

Parkinson's Disease, a slowly progressive disorder of the central nervous system. It is characterized by tremor in muscles that are at rest, and by stiffness and slowness of movement. The exact cause of the disease in most cases is unknown. Among the known causative factors are: arteriosclerosis, cerebral vascular accidents, head injuries, syphilis, toxic agents, and drugs.
Many research people are convinced that part of the basal ganglia is the brain center for much of the tremor and stiffness of Parkinson's disease.
Parkinson's disease is slightly more common in men than women and generally occurs between ages fifty and sixty. An extreme variability characterizes the rate

of development of this disease. For some, the onset of symptoms is mild, such as a slight tremor and stiffness on one side that does not impair functioning. For others the symptoms are marked, and within months of the onset the patient requires total care. There is a typical general appearance of the patient with Parkinson's disease: masklike and waxen features, rhythmic tremor of the fingers, stooped posture, and a gait in which the patient walks as if he were about to fall on his face. There may be drooling or a blank facial expression. This results from the loss of semiautomatic movements such as swallowing saliva and the movement of facial muscles. There is no cure for Parkinson's disease, but three kinds of treatment will help relieve symptoms. These are medication, physical therapy, and surgery. Stress and anxiety should be avoided as well as excitement, which causes the tremor to become worse.

Paronychia, infection of the tissues at the base of a nail.

Paroniria, frightful dreams.

Paropsis, disorder of vision.

Parorexia, craving for special foods.

Parosmia, smelling imaginary odors.

Parotid, located near the ear.

Parotid Gland, large salivary gland located over the jaw in front of the ear.

Parotitis, inflammation of the parotid gland, a large salivary gland.

Parous, having given birth to one or more children.

Parovarian, beside the ovary.

Paroxysm, sudden attack or recurrency of

Paroxysmal Tachycardia, a period of rapid heart beats that begins and ends suddenly.

Pars, pl., **Partes,** a part.

Particulate, composed of minute particles.

Parturient, giving birth; labor.

Parturifacient, medicine which speeds up birth.

Parturition, childbirth.

Paruria, any abnormality in excretion of urine.

Passion, strong emotion.

Pasteurization, method of sterilizing foods.

Patch Test, test carried out to determine sensitivity.

Patella, knee-cap.

Patency, state of being open, e.g., ducts, hollow tubes.

Patent Ductus Arteriosus, a congenital heart defect. A small duct between the artery leaving the left side of the heart (the aorta) and the artery leaving the right side of the heart (the pulmonary artery) which normally closes soon after birth, remains open.

Patent Medicine, remedy for public use obtained without prescription.

Patent, open.

Pathetic, pertaining to the feelings.

Pathic, pertaining to disease.

Pathogens, anything capable of producing disease.

Pathogenic, pertaining to the ability to produce disease.

Pathogenesis, the chain of events leading to the development of a disease.

Pathognomonic, a symptom that is so specific or so characteristic of a particular disease or disorder that a definite diagnosis is possible from its presence.

Pathology, study of diseases for their own interest, rather than directly with an immediate view to curing them.

Pathomania, abnormal wish to commit crime.

Pathophobia, extreme fear of disease.

Pathophoresis, communication of disease.

Patient, one under medical care.

Patulous, open; exposed.

Paunch, protruding abdomen.

Pavor, fear; fright.

Peccant, unhealthy.

Pectinate, like teeth of comb.

Pectoral, pertaining to the chest.

Pectus, chest; breast.

Pectus Carination, "Chicken breast."

Pedal, pertaining to the foot.

Pederasty, sexual intercourse through the anus.

Pediatrician, specialist in diseases of children.

Pediatrics, branch of medicine dealing with the diseases of children and their cure.

Pediatrist, pediatrician.

Pedicular, infested with lice.

Pediculicide, agent which kills lice.

Pediculosis, infestation of the scalp or hairy parts of the body or of clothing with lice. Lice are transmitted by direct contact with infected persons or their personal possessions, particularly clothing or infected bedding. The symptoms of pediculosis are inflammation of the skin, itching, and white eggs (nits) on the hair. The treatment consists of dusting the body and clothing (especially along the seams) with a specially prescribed powder.

Pediculosis Capititis, head lice.

Pediophobia, extreme fear of children or dolls.

Pedodontics, branch of dentistry dealing with children.

Pedophila, abnormal fondness for children.

Peduncle, stalk or stem.

Pelada, patchy baldness.

Pelage, hair covering the body.

Pelagism, seasickness.

Pellagra, disease due to lack of vitamin B.

Pellet, small pill.

Pellicle, thin tissue; scum on a liquid.

Pellucid, translucent.

Pelvic Examination, an internal examination of the vagina. cervix, and uterus.

Pelvis, bony part of the body lying between the thighs and the abdomen.
The exact shape of the pelvis differs between men and women. The male pelvis is narrower and more compact than the female pelvis. The male pelvis is designed for strength and speed; the female pelvis is designed to support pregnancies.
The upper outer edges of the pelvis form the area known as the hip. A person whose weight is normal for his height will be able to feel the edges of the pelvis.

Pemphigus, one of the most severe and rare types of oral ulcerations. It is a recurrent disease involving the mouth and skin. There are three forms of this disease: pemphigus vulgaris, pemphigus vegetans, and pemphigus conjunctivae. The most common type that involves the mouth is pemphigus vulgaris. This form of the disease can be either acute and malignant or chronic and benign.

The onset of pemphigus is insidious. At first the blisters are not painful. The patient feels a sensation of dryness in his mouth and a slight pain or discomfort when eating hot or spicy food. He may also have difficulty swallowing. Next, bullae—large blisters—form on the lips, tongue, cheek, palate, or gums. Often these blisters are not seen, because they break easily, leaving a reddish erosion with ragged edges. It is after they break that the blisters become very itchy and painful. Salivation increases and is often tinged with blood.

In about three-fourths of the cases of pemphigus, blisters form first in the mouth. Lesions on the skin may not appear for several months, and sometimes they never appear. When they do appear, they form over the entire body—face, trunk, arms, and legs. These blisters are thin-walled and translucent and are filled with a yellow fluid. When they break, they form a foul, yellow membrane.

Another characteristic symptom is "Nikolsky's sign"—the top layer of skin can be rubbed off with slight pressure.

Treatment of pemphigus can only be palliative, because there is no known cure for this disease. Cortisone has been used to alleviate symptoms, and penicillin has been used to prevent secondary infection. Mild mouthwashes can help relieve pain in the mouth. Since the cause is unknown, treatment can be directed only to the manifestation of the disease.

Pendulous, heavy and loosely hanging.

Penicillin, an antibiotic discovered in 1928 by Sir Alexander Fleming.

Penicillinase, a drug employed in the treatment of penicillin reactions.

Penis, male sex organ.

Penitis, inflammation of the penis.

Pepo, pumpkin seed used in removal of tapeworm.

Pepsic, peptic.

Pepsin, ferment found in the gastric juice which helps in the breakdown of protein.

Peptic, pertaining to the digestive tract.

Peptic Ulcer, a noncancerous, crater-like sore (called an erosion) in the wall of the stomach or intestine. This ulcer erodes through the thin, inner mucous membrane lining and into the deeper muscular wall of the stomach or intestine. Peptic ulcers occur only in those regions of the gastrointestinal tract that are bathed by the digestive juices secreted by the stomach. These digestive juices contain hydrochloric acid and a protein-digesting enzyme called pepsin; hence the name "peptic ulcer." Almost all peptic ulcers occur either in the stomach itself or in the small intestine just below the stomach. Those in the first portion of the intestine, the duodenum, are called duodenal ulcers, and those in the stomach are called gastric ulcers.

Statistics suggest that a person who has one or more family members with ulcers is slightly more prone to develop an ulcer than someone from a family having no ulcer patients. In many cases this may be because of the anxiety-ridden environment in such a family. In general, the treatment of ulcers by a physician is directed toward decreasing the amount of acid or irritants that reach the ulcer and interfere with the normal healing process. Proper diet; emphasis on frequent, small feedings; the use of antacids and drugs; and relief of nervous tension are important ways of accomplishing this.

Peracidity, excessive acidity.

Per Anum, by anus.

Perception, awareness.

Percussion, striking body as an aid to physical examination and diagnosis.

Percutanteous, through the skin.

Perforating, piercing.

Perforation, opening or hole in any area of body.

Peri- (prefix), around; near.

Periorticular, surrounding a joint.

Perianal, situated around the anus.

Pericardiac, around the heart.

Pericarditis, inflammation of sac surrounding the heart.

Pericardium, sac surrounding the heart.

Pericolic, around the colon.

Pericytial, around a cell.

Perimetrium, covering tissue of the womb.

Perinephric, situated around the kidneys.

Perineum, area between the sex organs and the anus.

Periodicity, occurring at regular intervals.

Period of Gestation, period from conception to childbirth.

Periodontal, around a tooth.

Periodontal Disease, a disorder affecting the tissues and membranes surrounding the teeth.

There are several types of periodontal disease. In its early stages the most common type takes the form of gingivitis, or inflammation of the gums. This condition may develop into periodontitis (sometimes called pyorrhea), the chronic, destructive stage of the disease. It usually affects people over twenty-five years of age. A major cause of periodontal disease is tartar, or calculus, that forms along the gums. This results in swelling and inflammation. As the disease progresses, the gums become more inflamed and pull away from the teeth, creating pockets between the gums and the teeth. Germs and food particles become wedged in these pockets, create more inflammation, and set up a vicious circle.

As the disease worsens, the inflammation spreads, the pockets deepen, and pus forms in them. The infected gums ulcerate and bleed, and tissue damage increases. In the final stages, the bone that supports the teeth is attacked and destroyed. Unless the person receives treatment, the teeth loosen and eventually come out.

Once periodontal disease has begun treatment will depend on the stage of the disease. If it has not progressed far, treatment may consist only of removing hardened tartar from around and under the gums. If pockets have formed between the teeth and gums, they must often be removed surgically to prevent further impaction of food.

In its final stages, periodontal disease attacks the underlying tissue that supports the teeth. Treatment at this stage may involve bone and reconstructive surgery.

Perionchyia, inflammation of area around a fingernail or toenail.

Periosteum, tissue around bone through which bone is nourished.

Periostitis, inflammation of the membrane surrounding a bone.

Periotic, located around the ear.

Peripatetic, changing from place to place.

Peripheral Nervous System, the part of the central nervous system that is composed of the twelve pairs of cranial nerves and thirty-one pairs of spinal nerves stemming from the brain and the spinal cord, respectively. The cranial nerves include voluntary fibers going to the eye muscles, the salivary glands, the heart, the smooth muscles of the lungs, and the intestinal tract. The spinal nerves send fibers to all muscles of the trunk and extremities, the involuntary fibers going to smooth muscles and glands of the gastrointestinal tract, genitourinary system, and cardiovascular system.

Peripheral Resistance, the resistance offered by the arterioles (small arteries) and capillaries to the flow of blood from the arteries to the veins. An increase in peripheral resistance causes a rise in blood pressure.

Periphery, away from center or midline of body.

Perirenal, around the kidney.

Perirhinal, around the nose.

Perish, die; disintegrate.

Peristalsis, the normal movements of the intestines which move the food along the digestive tract.

Peritoneum, the smooth, transparent membrane that lines the abdominal cavity and part of the pelvic region. The peritoneum allows the organs in the area to move against each other with little or no friction.

Peritonitis, inflammation of the lining tissue of the abdominal cavity. Peritonitis is caused by microorganisms that infect the peritoneum. This may follow a perforated ulcer, a ruptured appendix, an unsterile operation, or an abdominal wound, for instance. The chief symptoms are intense pain and tenderness. Peritonitis can be very serious if not treated promptly with antibiotics.

Peritonsillar, around the tonsil.

Perivascular, around a vessel.

Pernicious, severe; fatal.

Pernicious Anemia, a form of chronic anemia characterized by disturbances of the gastrointestinal and neurological systems. The exact cause of pernicious anemia is unknown. The disease is the result of a deficiency in the gastric juices that permit the body to absorb vitamin B^{12}. The lack of B^{12} causes premature death of red blood cells, thereby reducing the capacity of the blood to carry oxygen to the tissues. The onset of anemia is insidious. Depending on the stage of the disease, a patient may have the following symptoms: loss of appetite, fatigue, lassitude, pallor, faintness, jaundice, sore tongue and mouth, diarrhea, digestive dis-

turbances, depression and irritability that may ulti-
mately lead to a psychosis, numbness and tingling of
the fingers, other neurological deficits, and shortness of
breath on exertion. Pernicious anemia cannot be cured.
It is controlled by adequate diet and injection of vitamin B^{12} every week. Lifelong treatment is required if
neurological crippling is to be prevented.

Pernio, chillblain.

Per Os, by mouth.

Per Rectum, by rectum.

Perseveration, repetitive statements or answers to ques-
tions.

Perspiration, fluid produced by body at surface of the skin
which helps to control body temperature.

Pertussis, whooping cough.

Pervert, one who practices abnormal behavior.

Pervigilium, abnormal wakefulness.

Pes, foot or footlike structure.

Pes Contortis, clubfoot.

Pes Planus, flatfoot.

Pessary, device used to hold uterus in proper position.

Pesticides, substances used to kill pests. The pests may be
weeds, insects, rats and mice, algae, nematodes
(worms), and other destructive forms of life. Pesticides
that are used only for killing insects are called
insecticides. Killing garden pests, ridding homes of
insects or rodents, and defleaing or delousing pets are
common household uses of pesticides. Guarding
people's health and protecting fruits, vegetables, and
forests are well-known commercial, agricultural, and
governmental uses of pesticides. Improperly used, pesticides can and do cause illness and even death to
human beings. To avoid improper use, it is very important that anyone who uses a pesticide understands its
purpose and properties. It is most essential to understand that pesticides, by necessity, are poisons. However, there is a great variation between the different
compounds in use as pesticides with regard to their
toxic hazard. A few materials are dangerous in the relatively small amounts that spraymen encounter by skin
contact and by breathing during their work. However,
most compounds have not produced occupational
poisoning. Accidental ingestion (swallowing) has been
responsible for most of the deaths from pesticides. In

addition to fear of accidental exposure, there is concern about possible long-term effects of pesticide contamination that may remain in the environment and—through air, soil, food, and water—may eventually adversely affect living things. The possible danger here is in inhaling or ingesting dangerous amounts through air, water, or food. This is why the Food and Drug Administration sets limits on the amount of pesticide residue that may safely remain on food crops at harvest and also polices our food supply to enforce these limits.

Pestiferous, causing pestilence.

Pestilence, epidemic of contagious disease.

Pestle, device used to break up drugs in pharmacy.

Petit Mal, type of epilepsy in which the attacks are relatively slight.

pH, concentration of hydrogen ion or acidity; Neutral = pH 7.

Phactis, inflammation of the eye lens.

Phacomatacia, soft cataract.

Phagocyte, absorbing cell.

Phalanges, bones of fingers.

Phalanx, one of the bones of the fingers or toes.

Phallectomy, amputation of the penis.

Phallic, concerning male sex organ.

Phallus, male sex organ.

Phanic, visible.

Phantom Limb, the sensation of feeling in a limb that has been amputated. This phenomenon is caused by the stimulation of nerves in the remaining part of the limb that had continued into the amputated part.

Pharm., pharmaceutical; pharmacy.

Pharmaceutical, pertaining to drugs.

Pharmacist, druggist.

Pharmacology, the science that deals with the study of drugs in all its aspects.

Pharmacopoeia, an official listing of drugs and drug standards. In this country, the U.S.P. (United States Pharmacopeia) is the legally accepted standard text.

Pharmacy, drug store.

Pharyngitis, inflammation of the pharynx.

Pharyngoscope, instrument for examining the throat.

Pharynx, membraneous tube extending from oral cavity to level of first part of esophagus.

Phatne, tooth socket.

Phenobarbital, barbiturate used to sedate or produce sleep.

Phenol, a strong antiseptic.

Phenolphthalein, purgative.

Phenylbutazone, a drug used in the treatment of arthritis and related disorders, such as gout and osteoarthritis. Phenylbutazone is very effective in treating many cases of these conditions. However, phenylbutazone can have many serious side effects (vomiting, diarrhea, insomnia, edema, anemia, etc.). Consequently, the drug is often used as a last resort, and even then it is used with great care.

Phimosis, excessive tightness of the foreskin of the penis.

Phlebitis, the inflammation of a vein. This often occurs in the leg and usually involves the formation of a blood clot in the inflamed vein. The danger of phlebitis is that the blood clot will move from the affected vein to another area of the body where it can cause more damage. If the blood clot reaches the heart or brain, it may cause death.
The usual treatment is to immobilize the affected region by putting the patient to bed. At the same time, the patient is frequently given an anticoagulant drug to help dissolve the blood clot.

Phlebosclerosis, hardening of a vein.

Phlebothrombosis, formation of a clot in a vein.

Phlebotomy, opening of a vein.

Phlegm, thick mucus from respiratory tract.

Phlegmatic, sluggish.

Phlogistic, inducing inflammation.

Phobia, an extreme fear.

Phonal, pertaining to the voice.

Phonetics, science of vocal sounds.

Photodynia, pain in the eyes due to intense light.

Photophobia, extreme fear of light.

Photosensitive, sensitive to light.

Phrenetic, maniacal.

Phrenic, pertaining to the diaphragm or mind.

Phrenitis, delirium.

Phrenology, study of the mind through the shape of the skull.

Phrenoplegia, paralysis of the diaphragm.

Phthisiology, study of tuberculosis.

Phthisis, tuberculosis.

Phylaxis, bodily defense against infection.

Phyma, skin tumor.

Physic, cathartic; art of medicine.

Physical Fitness, a measure of the body's strength, stamina, and flexibility. It is a reflection of the ability to work with vigor and pleasure, without undue fatigue, with energy left over for enjoying hobbies and recreational activities, and for meeting unforeseen emergencies Physical fitness is important for mental health as well as for physical health. It requires proper nutrition, adequate rest and relaxation, good sleeping habits, good health practices, and especially adequate physical exercise. The human body contains more than six hundred muscles; overall, the body is more than half muscle. Muscles make possible every overt motion. They also push food along the digestive tract, suck air into the lungs, and tighten blood vessels to raise blood pressure when more pressure is needed to meet an emergency. The heart itself is a muscular pump. Muscles are meant to be used. When they are not used, or are not used enough, they deteriorate. An obvious effect of regular exercise is the firming of flabby muscles. In addition, research indicates that exercise produces beneficial changes in the functioning of internal organs—especially the heart, lungs, and circulatory system. The heartbeat becomes stronger and steadier, breathing becomes deeper, and circulation improves.

Physician, licensed medical doctor.

Physics, study of natural forces and phenomena.

Physiogonomy, face.

Physiology, science which deals with the functions of the body.

Physique, body build.

Phytin, material from plants used as stimulants.

Phytotoxin, plant poison.

Pia, one of membranous coverings of brain and spinal cord.

Pica, an abnormal craving to eat odd things.

Picric Acid, a substance used in the treatment of minor burns.

Piedra, hair disease.

Pigment, coloring substance.

Pilary, pertaining to the hair.

Pileous, hairy.

Piles, enlarged, painful veins in the rectum or around the anus.

Pill, capsule containing medication.

Pillion, temporary artificial leg.

Pilonidal, cyst containing hairs, frequently found at the base of the spine.

Pilose, hairy.

Pilus, hair.

Pimple, small pointed area on skin, at times filled with infectious material.

Pineal Gland, small gland about the size of a pea in the lower part of the brain.

Pinquecula, thickened area on edge of cornea of eye.

Pinkeye, contagious eye inflammation; conjunctivitis.

Pinna, projecting part of external ear.

Pinpoint Vision, a defect of the eye in which there is vision in the center of the eye only, with no visual field at all.

Pinworm, parasite found in intestine and around anus. Pinworms enter the body when pinworm eggs are swallowed. The eggs hatch in the stomach, and the larvae pass through the small intestine into the large intestine. They remain there until they develop into adult worms, probably within five to six weeks. The female worms are then ready to deposit their eggs. They migrate down the rectum and out of the anus, where they deposit their eggs in the folds of skin surrounding the anus. After expelling many thousands of eggs, the female worm shrivels up and dies. The male worms may also migrate out of the anus and die. The migration and egg-laying usually occur at night, from a half hour to several hours after the person has gone to bed. In the case of heavy infections, migration may occur during the day, especially during periods of rest or relaxation. In the moist folds of the skin each egg develops to the infective stage in five to seven hours. The cycle of infection (or reinfection of the same individual) is completed when the infective eggs are swallowed. A sensation varying in intensity from a very mild tickling to severe itching or pain usually occurs when migrating female worms are on the anus or the surrounding skin. In women and girls, migrating worms may enter the vulva and vagina, frequently causing a vaginal discharge. Infected children sometimes have dark circles under the eyes and are pale. Restlessness, sleeplessness, loss of appetite, loss of weight, and sometimes nausea and vomiting occur. Infected children are apt to be irritable, hard to manage, and inattentive at school. Diagnosis of pinworm infection is based on finding the female worm or the pinworm eggs.

Pit, depression.

Pithecoid, apelike.

Pituita, phlegm.

Pituitarism, disorder of pituitary function.

Pituitary Gland, small gland at the base of the brain which affects all the other glands of the body.

Pityriasis, group of diseases in which the main symptom is a scaly skin.

Placebo, a harmless, inactive substance given to patients in controlled tests. The placebo helps the researcher to evaluate the effectiveness of the real drug by guarding against any psychological effects or reactions to the idea of the medication.
In many experiements, half the patients will be given the test drug and half will be given a placebo. The patients are not told whether they are taking the real drug or the placebo. The results are then tabulated to see if there is any difference. In a double-blind experiment neither the patients nor the physician are aware of who is getting the real drug.

Placenta, organ by which the unborn infant is attached to the inside of the womb and through which infants' body needs are supplied.
Blood from the fetus flows in and out through two arteries and a vein. These arteries and the vein are encased in the umbilical cord, which attaches to the surface of the placenta at one end and to the baby's navel at the other end. The waste products of the fetus are carried through the blood vessels of the umbilical cord into the placenta, where they are exchanged for oxygen and nutrients from the mother. The vein in the cord carries these materials back to the baby. The main pur-

pose of the placenta is to make possible this interchange. Once the baby is born, the placenta is no longer needed. After birth the placenta starts to separate from its attachment to the lining of the uterus.

Plague, epidemic disease transmitted by fleas of rats. There are two major types of plague: bubonic plague and pneumonic plague. Pneumonic plague attacks the lungs; bubonic plague causes buboes, or swollen lymph glands.

Planocyte, wandering cell.

Planta, sole of the foot.

Plantar, pertaining to the sole of the foot.

Plantar Wart, painful wart occurring on the bottom of the foot.

Plaque, any patch or accumulation. Plaques play a major role in atherosclerosis, or hardening of the arteries, and in tooth decay and periodontal disease.

Plasma, colorless fluid part of the blood as distinct from blood cells.

Plaster of Paris, a chemical substance used to make hard casts for the immobilization of injured body parts.

Plastic, pertaining to plastic surgery; moldable; any material that can be molded.

Plastic Surgery, a special branch of surgery that is concerned with correcting disfigurements. Plastic surgery includes purely cosmetic surgery, such as restructuring unattractive noses. However, plastic surgery is also concerned with the reduction of scar tissue. This can be extremely important, because large scars (as from extensive burns) can cause a loss of mobility. The major aim of the plastic surgeon is to reduce the amount of the scar tissue to the smallest possible size. This is frequently achieved by hiding the scar within natural wrinkles.

Platelet, small disc in blood stream used for blood coagulation.

Platycrania, flattening of the skull.

Platypodia, flat foot.

Pledget, small piece of gauze soaked in antiseptic.

Pleonemia, increased amount of blood in a part.

Pleonexia, extreme greediness.

Plethora, abnormal amount of blood.

Pleura, thin tissue covering the lungs and lining the interior walls of the chest cavity.

Pleurisy, an inflammation of the pleura, the membrane that covers the lungs. The most common cause of pleurisy is infection, either viral or bacterial. Dry pleurisy is the easiest type of pleurisy to diagnose. There is sudden pain, usually during respiration. The pain is caused by the friction that results when the two layers of the pleura rub together. In cases of dry pleurisy, the protective fluid between the two pleura layers is partially replaced by a sticky substance known as fibrin. Dry pleurisy is not contagious, although the underlying cause may be. It is treated by any drugs needed to stop the infection and by bed rest. Frequently, drugs are not needed at all. Serofibrinous pleurisy, or pleurisy with effusion, is caused by an excess accumulation of fluid between the two layers of the pleura. Treatment may include the withdrawal of the excess fluid through a long needle inserted into the space between the pleura layers. Empyema is a type of pleurisy in which fluid containing pus infiltrates the area between the pleura membranes.

Pleurodynia, pain in the muscles between the ribs.

Plexor, percussion hammer.

Plexus, groups of nerves, lymphatic glands or blood vessels in the body.

Plica, fold.

Plug, obstruction.

Plumbism, lead poisoning.

Plummer-Vinson Syndrome, a wasting-away of the mucous membranes of the mouth, pharynx, and esophagus. This syndrome is caused by deficiencies in the diet and frequently precedes cancer of the mouth. It is common among women in Sweden and apparently accounts for there unusually high incidence of mouth cancer.

PMS (premenstrual syndrome), condition occurring from one to two weeks prior to a woman's normal menstrual period. Symptoms include nervousness, fatigue, and depression, as well as breast tenderness, water retention, headache, and general aches.

Pneumatic, pertaining to respiration.

Pneumococcus, germ which can attack the body, usually the lungs.

Pneumonectomy, surgical removal of a lung.

Pneumonia, a general term for infection of the lungs. It can be caused by different kinds of bacteria or virus or by the presence of foreign matter such as fatty droplets of liquids that have been inhaled. Frequently, the symptoms of pneumonia include high fever, chills, vomiting, and a cough. Difficult, rapid breathing is another symptom.

Pneumonia begins when the microbes or the foreign matter that has entered the lungs sets up an inflammation. As part of the inflammation, fluid rushes into the lungs. When the cause of the disease is a virus or bacteria, the fluid is used by the invading organisms as a culture, or growth media. When the cause is foreign matter, the fluid provides a growing place for any organisms already present in the lungs or respiratory system. Pneumonia can be classified by the causative agent or by the location of the infection.

Pneumonopathy, any lung disease.

Pneumorrhagia, lung hemorrhage.

Pneumothorax, abnormal entrance of air or gas into lung sacs, causing an imbalance of pressures and difficult respiration.

Pock, pustule.

Podagra, gout affecting foot.

Podalgia, pain in the feet.

Podiatrist, specialist in foot ailments.

Pogoniasis, excessive beard growth.

Point, tiny spot or area.

Pointillage, massage with the finger tips.

Poison, any substance that causes bodily disturbance, injury, or death by chemical rather than mechanical means. The action of a poison depends on several factors. The action will be more severe if a large dose is taken, because more of the poison will be absorbed in a short period of time. The toxicity of substances varies greatly—a few drops of one poison might be immediately fatal, while another poison might not be harmful unless taken by the tablespoonful. The age and body weight of the victim should also be considered. Infants, young children, and very old people are more likely to be killed by small doses of poison. In general, the less a person weighs, the smaller will be the fatal dose. Another factor that influences the action of poisons taken by mouth is the condition of the stomach;

poisons taken on an empty stomach will act much more quickly (and therefore more violently) than those taken when the stomach is full.

The action of any poison is dependent, also, on the tolerance that the individual has for the particular substance. Some people seem to have a natural resistance to the action of certain poisons; others are so highly sensitive to them that even a small amount, such as might be given in a medicine, produces toxic effects. Habit is sometimes a factor to consider—drug addicts can tolerate doses of the habit-forming drugs that might kill the average person. The effectiveness of a poison also depends on the general health of the victim. The physical state of the poisonous substance also determines its effectiveness. Gases are absorbed more quickly than liquids, and liquids are absorbed more quickly than solids. Related to this is the fact that the way in which a poison enters the body determines to some extent the speed and effectiveness with which it acts. In general, inhaled poisons are likely to work most quickly, injected poisons next, and poisons taken by mouth more slowly. Poisoning by skin contact usually occurs quite slowly over an extended period of time. Also, some substances are poisonous when taken in one way but not when taken in another; for example, snake venom may cause death when injected (as by a snakebite) but may be relatively harmless if swallowed.

Poisoning, ingestion of substance toxic to body.

Poison Ivy, a poisonous plant. It grows in the form of climbing vines, shrubs that trail on the ground, and erect shrubbery growing without support.

The leaves vary in length from one to four inches. They are green and glossy in summer; in the spring and fall they are red or russet. The fruit is white and waxy and resembles mistletoe. Although poison ivy assumes many forms and displays seasonal changes in leaf coloring, it has one constant characteristic that makes it easy to recognize: the leaves always grow in clusters of three. The irritating substance in poison ivy is the oily sap in the leaves, flowers, fruit, stem, bark, and roots. The plant is poisonous even after long drying, but is particularly irritating in the spring and early summer when it is full of sap. Most cases of ivy poisoning are caused by direct contact with the plant. Some are caused by handling clothing, garden implements, and pets that have been contaminated by the oily sap.

Poitrinaire, one having a chronic chest disease.

Poliomyelitis (Infantile Paralysis),•a disease caused by any one of three closely related ciruses. Poliomyelitis is best known as a disease that causes paralysis. However, only the most severe form of polio (as poliomyelitis is sometimes called) causes lasting paralysis. The great majority of cases result in no lasting paralysis.
The virus causing poliomyelitis enters the body through the respiratory 'system. The virus attacks the cells in the central nervous system. The exact method by which the virus cells move from the respiratory system to the central nervous system is not known.

Poliosis, absence of hair coloring.

Pollen, male sex cells of plants.

Pollex, thumb or big toe.

Pollinosis, hay fever.

Pollution, making impure; discharge of semen without sexual intercourse.

Polyarthritis, inflammation of several joints.

Polycholia, excessive bile secretion.

Polyclinic, medical center treating many diseases.

Polycyesis, pregnancy with more than one fetus.

Polycythemia, condition in which there is an excess of red blood cells.

Polycytosis, excess of blood cells.

Polydactylism, having more than five fingers or five toes.

Polydipsia, excessive desire to drink.

Polyemia, excessive blood in the body.

Polyglandular, affecting many glands.

Polygraph, an instrument for simultaneously recording several different pulsations.

Polygyny, marriage to more than one woman at one time.

Polyhedral, many sides.

Polymenorrhea, unusual frequency of menstruation.

Polymyositis, inflammation of many muscles.

Polyneural, pertaining to many nerves.

Polyneuritis, inflammation of more than one group of nerves.

Polyp, outgrowths in the nose, intestines or bladder.

Polypathia, having more than one disease at a time.

Polyphagia, excessive eating.

Polyplegia, paralysis of several muscles.

Polypus, polyp.

Polyunsaturated fat, a fat so constituted chemically that it is capable of absorbing additional hydrogen. These fats are usually liquid oils of vegetable origin, such as corn oil or safflower oil. A diet with a high polyunsaturated fat content tends to lower the amount of cholesterol in the blood. These fats are sometimes substituted for saturated fat in a diet in an effort to lessen the hazard of fatty deposits in the blood vessels.

Polyuria, excessive urination.

Pons, a part of the brain which bridges several other sections of the nervous system.

Pontic, false tooth.

Popliteal, pertaining to the back of the leg and the bend of the knee.

Pore, small opening in skin or tissue.

Porous, having many pores.

Porrigo, ringworm.

Portio, part.

Portio Dura, facial nerve.

Porus, pore.

Position, placement of the body.

Positive, affirmative; indicating the presence of a disorder.

Posology, system of dosage.

Postcibal, after eating.

Postcoital, after sexual intercourse.

Postepileptic, after an epileptic attack.

Posterior, behind; at the back part.

Posthetomy, circumsion.

Posthumous, after death.

Postmortem, autopsy; after death.

Postnasal, situated behind the nose.

Postnasal Drip, relatively constant nasal discharge which drips or drains down the throat.

Postnatal, immediately after birth.

Postoperative, happening after an operation.

Postoral, in the back of the mouth.

Postpartum, after childbirth.

Postprandial, after a meal.

Postpubescent, after puberty.

Posture, the position of the body. Good posture is the correct alignment of the body and all body parts when standing, sitting, lying down, or in any phase of activity. Good posture helps to conserve energy, promotes the efficient use of muscles, and avoids back strain and fatigue.

Postuterine, behind the uterus.

Potable, adequate for drinking.

Potamophobia, extreme fear of large bodies of water.

Potency, strength; ability to perform coitus.

Potion, dose of liquid medicine.

Pouch, pocket-like cavity.

Poultice, hot, moist mass to be placed on the skin.

Pox, blisters and scars on the skin caused by certain diseases.

Practice, professional diagnosis and treatment of disease.

Practitioner, physician.

Pragmatagnosia, inability to recognize objects.

Prandial, pertaining to a meal.

Precordia, area overlying heart.

Pregnancy, state of being with child.

Pregravidic, preceding pregnancy.

Prehensile, able to grasp.

Prehension, grasping.

Preictal, preceding a stroke or attack.

Prelingual Deafness, the total or near-total loss of hearing that occurs before normal speech habits have been established. The lack of meaningful hearing during infancy and early childhood (when speech develops) has drastic effects on the development of both speech and language. Normally, speech develops as a direct result of hearing. Speech is both a way of making the sounds that are called words and a system of symbols that stand for something. Language is the system of symbols that uses words to represent objects, actions, ideas, and meanings.
The small child who cannot hear is doubly handicapped. He has difficulty acquiring the meanings for which language stands as well as difficulty in talking.

Premature, born before maturity.

Premature Infant, one weighing less than 5.5 pounds at birth.

Premenstrual, preceding menstruation.

Premonitary, warning.

Premunition, immunization by vaccination.

Prenatal, before birth.

Preoral, in front of the mouth.

Prepuce, foreskin of penis.

Presbyatry, treatment of diseases of the aged.

Presbyacusia, partial loss of hearing in old age.

Presbyopia, loss of elasticity in eyes which occurs in old age.

Prescription, written order for drug authorized by a physician.

Pressor, a substance that raises the blood pressure and accelerates the heartbeat.

Pressure, stress; strain.

Pressure Point, a place where a main artery lies near the skin surface and over a bone.

Preventive, prophylactic.

Priapism, continued erection of the penis without sexual desire.

Prickly Heat, irritations of the skin in which blisters form due to increased temperature.

Primary, principal.

Primary Hypertension, an elevated blood pressure that is not caused by kidney or other evident disease.

Primigravida, woman in her first pregnancy.

Primipara, woman who has given birth once.

Primitive, original.

Primordial, primitive.

Princeps, primary artery.

Principal, most important.

Probe, instrument for exploring the interior of the body.

Procaine, a drug used as a local anesthetic; better known as novocaine.

Proconceptive, aiding conception.

Procreate, to beget children.

Proctalgia, pain in the rectum.

Proctitis, inflammation of the rectum or anus.

Proctology, branch of medicine concerned with the rectum.

Proctoscope, an instrument used to examine the rectum.

Proctoscopy, examination of the rectum.

Procumbent, prone.

Prodrome, early symptoms of impending illness.

Progeny, offspring.

Progeria, condition causing early aging.

Progesterone, an important female hormone.

Prognathism, having projecting jaws.

Prognosis, medical name for the outlook of a disease.

Proiota, sexual precocity.

Prolapse, abnormal position of internal organ.

Proliferation, multiplication of cells.

Prominence, projection; elevation.

Prone, lying face downward.

Prootic, in front of the ear.

Propagation, reproduction.

Prophylactic, preventing disease.

Prophylaxis, prevention of disease.

Pro Re Nata, according to circumstances.

Prorrhaphy, advancement.

Prosodemic, spread from one person to another.

Prosopospasm, facial spasm.

Prostate, small gland in the male situated at the base of the bladder, concerned with preparation of the semen.

Prostatitis, inflammation of the prostate gland.

Prosthesis, substitute for missing part.

Prosthetics, branch of surgery dealing with artificial parts.

Prostigmine Test, a test for pregnancy.

Prostitution, having sexual relations for profit or gain.

Prostration, exhaustion.

Protein, the basic substance of every cell in the body.

Prothrombin, chemical substance important in blood coagulation.

Protistology, microbiology.

Protoplasm, prime material in living organism.

Protozoa, microscopic, one-celled organisms.

Protraction, the act of moving a part forward.

Protuberance, projection.

Provisional, of temporary use.

Proximate, nearest.

Pruritus, itching.

Prussiate, cyanide.

Psellism, stuttering.

Pseudocrisis, false crisis.

Pseudocyesis, imaginary pregnancy with some physical findings of the condition.

Psittacosis, disease spread by parrots, love-birds, canaries and other birds kept as pets.

Psoriasis, chronic skin disease in which red scaly patches develop.

Psychanalysis, psychoanalysis.

Psyche, mind.

Psychectampsia, acute mania.

Psychiatrist, one who specializes in psychiatry.

Psychiatry, study and treatment of mental disorders.

Psychic, pertaining to the mind.

Psychics, psychology.

Psychoanalysis, method of obtaining a patient's past emotional history.

Psychocoma, mental stupor.

Psychogenesis, mental development.

Psychognosis, study of mental and emotional activity.

Psychology, science dealing with mental functions.

Psychopath, one who has no sense of moral obligation.

Psychopathy, any mental disorder.

Psychophylaxis, mental hygiene.

Psychosis, type of insanity in which one loses almost complete touch with reality.

Psychosomatic Disease, physical ailments due to emotional causes.

Psychotherapy, treatment of mental and emotional disorders.

Ptarmic, causing sneezing.

Ptarmus, sneezing.

Ptomaine, specific poisoning caused by putrified food.

Ptosis, drooping of the upper eyelid.

Ptyalism, excess secretion of saliva.

Ptyalorrhea, excessive secretion of saliva.
Ptysis, spitting.

Puberal, pertaining to puberty.

Puberty, period of rapid growth and development between childhood and adult life.

Pubes, hairy area above the genitals.

Pubis, bone at front of pelvis.

Pudenda, the external sex organ.

Pudic, pudendal.

Puerile, pertaining to a child.

Puerilism, childishness.

Puerpera, woman who has had a child.

Puerperium, period immediately following childbirth.

Pulmonary, pertaining to the lungs.

Pulmonary Artery, the large artery that conveys unoxygenated blood from the lower right chamber of the heart to the lungs.

Pulmonic, pulmonary.

Pulpalgia, pain in the pulp of a tooth.

Pulpy, soft.

Pulsation, rhythmic throb.

Pulse Pressure, the difference between the blood pressure in the arteries when the heart is in contraction (systole) and when it is in relaxation (diastole).

Pulso, pressure variation in arteries due to action of heart; can be felt where arteries are close to skin.

Pulsus, pulse.

Pulsus Alternans, a pulse in which there is a regular alternation of weak and strong beats.

Pulverulent, powdery.

Punctum, point.

Punctum Caecum, blind spot.

Puncture, pierce.

Pupil, part of eye which opens or closes to adjust to light or object.

Pupillary, pertaining to the pupil.

Purgative, drug to relieve constipation.

Purge, to evacuate the bowels by medicine.

Purkinje Fibers, the specialized fibers that form a network in the walls of the lower chambers of the heart.

Purpura, purple areas or bruises on body due to abnormal blood clotting.

Purulent, forming or containing pus.

Pus, product of infection containing dead cell and cell debris.

Pustule, pimple.

Pyarthrosis, pus in a joint cavity.

Pyelitis, inflammation of the pelvis of the kidney, that is, the area where the kidney is connected to the ureter, the tube leading down to the bladder.

Pyemia, form of blood poisoning in which the germs are carried in the blood and produce abscesses.

Pygal, pertaining to the buttocks.

Pyknemia, thickening of the blood.

Pyloric Stenosis, an obstruction in the digestive system.

Pylorus, valve which lies at one end of the stomach and controls the entry of food into the small intestine.

Pyocele, pus around the testis.

Pyocolpos, pus in the vagina.

Pyocyst, sac of pus in body.

Pyoderma, any skin inflammation that produces pus.

Pyogenesis, formation of pus.

Pyorrhea, infection of the gums which causes the edges of the tooth sockets to bleed easily when teeth are being brushed.

Pyretic, pertaining to fever.

Pyretolysis, lowering of fever.

Pyrexia, increased body temperature, high fever.

Pyrogenic, causing fever.

Pyromania, obsessive compulsion to start fires.

Pyrophobia, extreme fear of fire.

Pyrosis, burning pain in stomach; acid taste in mouth.

Pyrotic, burning.

Pyuria, pus in urine.

— Q —

Q Fever, a disease caused by microorganisms called rickettsiae.

Quack, a faker in medical science.

Quadripara, woman giving birth to her fourth child.

Quadriplegia, paralysis of arms and legs.

Quadruplets, a pregnancy that results in the birth of four babies.

Quarantine, enforced isolation of people suffering from an infectious disease.

Quartan Fever, a type of malaria in which the patient has malarial symptoms every fourth day (counting the day the symptoms occur as the first day.)

Quassation, shattering.

Quickening, the feeling of life of a baby by a pregnant woman.

Quinidine, a drug that is occasionally used to treat abnormal rhythms of the heartbeat.

Quinine, drug used in the treatment of malaria.

Quinsy, formation of an abscess around one of the tonsils.

Quintan, every fifth day.

Quintipara, woman giving birth to her fifth child.

Rabbeting, interlocking of the splintered edges of a fractured bone.

Rabbit Fever, virus disease transmitted by eating or handling infected animals; tularemia.

Rabiate, one who has rabies.

Rabic, pertaining to rabies.

Rabid, pertaining to rabies.

Rabies, a fatal disease of man affecting the brain and spinal cord if untreated.

Race, class of people of similar inheritance and ethnic qualities.

Rachialgia, pain in spine.

Rachianalgesia, spinal anesthesia.

Rachicentesis, puncture into spinal canal.

Rachidian, pertaining to the spine.

Rachiocampsis, curvature of the spine.

Rachiodynia, painful condition of spinal column.

Rachis, spinal column.

Rachisschisis, spinal column fissure; congenital opening.

Rachitec, pertaining to rickets.

Radiation, rays that in proper dosage can be used to treat certain diseases.

Radicular, pertaining to a root.

Radiculitis, inflammation of a nerve root.

Radiectomy, removal of the root of a tooth.

Radioactivity, emitting of penetrating rays or small particles.

Radiograph, an x-ray film.

Radiography, taking of x-rays.

Radiologist, medical specialist who uses radiation for diagnosis and treatment.

Radiology, branch of medicine using radiant energy in diagnosis and treatment of disease.

Radiolus, sound; probe.

Radiotherapeutic, use of x-ray or radium for treatment.

Radium, an intensely radioactive metallic element.

Radius, short arm bone extending from elbow to wrist.

Radix, root.

Rale, abnormal sound coming from air passages of lungs.

Rami, branch.

Ramify, to branch.

Ramitis, inflammation of a nerve root.

Ramollissement, morbid softening of some organ or tissue.

Ramus, branch of an artery, vein or nerve; branchlike part.

Rancid, offensive; sour.

Range of Accommodation, difference between the least and greatest distance of clear vision.

Ranula, swelling under the tongue due to the blocking of a salivary gland.

Rape, sexual intercourse without consent of female.

Rash, skin eruption.

Raspatory, surgical file.

Rasura, Rasure, scraping; shaving.

Rat, rodent frequently used in experiments.

Rat Bite Fever, an infectious disease passed to human beings by bite of an infected animal.

Ratio, proportion.

Ration, fixed portion of food and drink for a certain period.

Rational, according to reason.

Rationalization, making an irrational thing appear reasonable.

Rattle, rale.

Rattle, Death, gurgling sound heard in the trachea of the dying.

Rauwolfia, drug which lowers blood pressure and causes relaxation in mind and body.

Rave, talk irrationally.

Ravish, rape.

Raw Milk, milk that has not been pasteurized.

Raynaud's Disease, circulatory disturbance affecting extremities.

R.C.P., Royal College of Physicians.

R.C.S., Royal College of Surgeons.

Re- (prefix), back; again.

Reaction, response.

Recall, memory.

Receptaculum, vessel or cavity which contains fluid.

Receptor, a nerve ending that is sensitive to stimuli.

Recessus, small hollow or recess.

Recidivation, recurrence of a disease.

Recipe, prescription; formula.

Recipient, one who receives a thing.

Recline, lie down.

Reconstituent, an agent which strengthens a part of the body by replacing lost material.

Recrement, secretion which is reabsorbed into the body after performing its function.

Recrudescence, reappearance of symptoms of a disease.

Rectal, pertaining to the rectum.

Rectal Reflex, normal desire to evacuate feces.

Rectalgia, rectal pain.

Rectectomy, surgical removal of the rectum or anus.

Rectified, made pure or straight.

Rectitis, inflammation of the rectum.

Rectoclysis, gradual introduction of fluid into rectum.

Rectocolitis, inflammation of the rectum and colon.

Rectostenosis, stricture of the rectum.

Rectostomy, making an artificial opening into the rectum to relieve stricture.

Rectum, lowest six inches of the intestinal tract adjoining the anus.

Rectus, straight; any straight muscle.

Recumbent, lying down.

Recuperation, restoration to health.

Recurrent, reappearing.

Recurve, bend backward.

Red Blood Cell, blood corpuscle containing hemoglobin.

Redressment, correction of a deformity; dressing a wound a second time or more.

Red Softening, hemorrhagic softening of brain and spinal cord.

Reduce, decrease.

Reduction, restoration to normal position.

Reduction Diet, diet which eliminates fat producing foods.

Reduplicated, folded back on itself.

Referred Pain, pain felt in part of the body other than its source.

Refine, purify.

Reflex, an involuntary action caused by a stimulus to the nerves.

Reflexogenic, causing a reflex action.

Reflux, backward flow.

Refracta Dosi, in divided doses.

Refraction, eye testing to determine amount of vision.

Refractory, not easily treated.

Refracture, break again.

Refrangible, capable of refraction.

Refresh, renew, revive.

Refrigerant, medicine which relieves thirst and reduces fever.

Refusion, return flow of blood to the vessels.

Regeneration, regrowth or repair of part of body.

Regimen, course of therapy to improve health.

Region, particular body area.

Registry, placement bureau for nurses.

Regression, process of going back to a prior status in physical or mental illness.

Regressive, subsiding, reverting.

Regular, normal.

Regurgitant, backward flow.

Regurgitate, to vomit.

Rehabilitation, restoration to activity of a handicapped person.

Rehalation, rebreathing.

Reichman's Disease, constant excessive gastric secretion.

Reinfection, return of infection.

Reimplantation, replacement of a part to its original location.

Rejuvenation, return to a youthful or normal state.

Relapse, recurrence of an illness.

Relapsing Fever, an infectious disease in which periods of fever alternate with periods of normal temperature.

Relaxant, agent which lessens tension or loosens bowels.

Relaxation, reduction of tension.

Remak's Axis Cylinder, conducting part of a nerve.

Remedial, curative.

Remedy, substance that is used in treatment of disease.

Remission, abatement.

Ren, the kidney.

Renal, pertaining to the kidney.

Renal Circulation, the circulation of the blood through the kidneys.

Renal Pelvis, the cavity in the middle of a kidney; it is the upper end of the ureter.

Renifieur, one who is sexually stimulated by certain odors, especially that of urine.

Reniform, kidney-shaped.

Rennin, a prominent component of gastric juices during infancy. It helps to coagulate milk protein.

Repair, replace; heal.

Repellent, reducing swelling; that which repels insects.

Repletion, full; satisfied; fullness of blood; plethora.

Reportable Diseases, diseases which must be reported to public health authorities.

Reposition, act of replacing a part.

Repositor, instrument for replacing a part.

Repression, suppression into unconsciousness of unacceptable ideas and emotion.

Reproduction, begetting of offspring.

Resection, excision of part of body tissue.

Reserpine, drug used to lower blood pressure.

Residue, that which remains after removal of a part.

Residuum, residue.

Resilience, elasticity.

Resilient, elastic.

Resistance, ability to protect self from disease.

Resolution, subsiding of an inflammation.

Respirable, suitable for respiration.

Respiration, breathing.

Respirator, mechanical device used to aid breathing.

Respiratory, pertaining to respiration.

Respiratory System, the parts of the body that together are responsible for bringing air into the lungs and for expelling carbon dioxide from the body.

Rest, period of inactivity.

Restiform, ropelike; rope-shaped.

Restitution, restoring.

Restorative, promoting health; remedy.

Restraint, forcible control.

Resuscitation, artificial respiration which is used to restore breathing after drowning, electric shock or other conditions interfering with breathing.

Resuscitator, mechanical device used for artificial respiration.

Retardation, delay.

Retarded Depression, depressed state of manic depressive psychosis.

Retching, unsatisfactory attempt to vomit.

Rete, network.

Retention, holding back.

Retention Cyst, cyst caused by retention of a secretion in a gland.

Retention of Urine, failure to urinate.

Reticular, netlike.

Reticulation, formation of a network mass.

Reticulum, network in cells.

Retina, part of the eye that receives the image and which is connected to the brain by the optic nerve.

Retinal, pertaining to the retina.

Retinitis, inflammation of the retina, the innermost coat of the eye.

Retinitis Pigmentosa, a disease, frequently hereditary, marked by progressive pigmentation and deterioration of the retina and disturbance of its nerve elements.

Retinosis, degeneration of the retina.

Retractile, able to be drawn back.

Retraction, drawing back.

Retractor, surgical instrument used to hold back the edges of an incision.

Retrocolic, behind the colon.

Retrocollic, pertaining to the back of the neck.

Retroinfection, infection transmitted by the fetus to the mother.

Retrolingual, behind the tongue.

Retronasal, behind the nose.

Retroposed, displaced backward.

Revulsant, causing transfer of disease or blood from one part of body to another; agent which draws blood to inflamed site.

Reye's Syndrome, serious and often fatal childhood complication that follows viral infections, influenza, and chicken pox which have been treated with aspirin. Symptoms appear a few days after the child has recovered from the viral illness and include: vomiting, drowsiness, lethargy, a change in mental status such as forgetfulness or disorientation, loss of consciousness, convulsions, and coma. There is no cure.

Rhachis, spinal column.

Rhagades, skin cracks.

-rhagia, (suffix), bleeding.

Rhegma, rupture, fracture, tear.

Rheum, watery discharge.

Rheumatalgia, rheumatic pain.

Rheumatic Fever, disease affecting joints, skin and sometimes the heart; believed due to an allergic reaction to specific bacteria.

Rheumatic Heart Disease, the damage done to the heart, particularly the heart valves, by one or more attacks of rheumatic fever.

Rheumatism, pain, swelling and deformity of joints of unknown cause.

Rheumatoid, of the nature of rheumatism.

Rhexis, rupture of a blood vessel or organ.

Rh. Factor, a substance found in the red blood cells; about 15% of people do not have this factor and are therefore called RH negative.

Rhinal, pertaining to the nose.

Rhinalgia, nasal pain.

Rhinesthesia, sense of smell.

Rhinitis, inflammation of the lining of the nose.

Rhinobyon, nasal plug.

Rhinocleisis, nasal obstruction.

Rhinodynia, nasal pain.

Rhinolalia, nasal voice quality.

Rhinologist, nose specialist.

Rhinology, branch of medicine dealing with the nose.

Rhinopathy, any nasal disease.

Rhinophyma, disease of the nose in which it becomes greatly enlarged.

Rhinoplasty, plastic or cosmetic surgery to remodel the nose.

Rhinorrhagia, nosebleed.

Rhinotomy, surgical incision of the nose.

Rhodocyte, red blood cell.

Rhodopsin, a red pigment located in the rods of the eye.

Rhoncus, rale; rattling sound in chest.

Rhypophagy, eating of filth.

Rhypophobia, extreme fear of filth.

Rhythm, measured time or movement; noting the periods of fertility and sterility in the female during the menstrual cycle.

Rhytidosis, wrinkling of skin or cornea.

Rib, bone and cartilage that form the chest cavity and protects its contents.

Ribosomes, large particles containing RNA. Ribosomes are found in the cytoplasm of a cell.

Ribs, False, five ribs on each side not directly attached to sternum.

Ribs, Floating, two lower ribs not attached to sternum.

Rickets, this is a disease caused by lack of vitamin D.

Ridge, narrow, elevated border.

Rigidity, stiffness.

Rigor, chill preceding a fever; rigidity.

Rigor Mortis, stiffening of muscles after death.

Rima, crack.

Rimula, minute crack.

Rind, skin or cortex of an organ or person.

Ringworm, fungus infection.

Risus, laugh; grin.

Ritter's Disease, severe skin inflammation seen in infants.

R.N., registered nurse.

RNA, single-strand molecules of a type of nucleic acid. RNA is the abbreviation for ribonucleic acid.

Roborant, tonic; strengthening.

Rocky Mountain Spotted Fever, infectious disease characterized by fever, pains in bone and muscle and reddish eruptions.

Rodent Ulcer, small, hard skin ulcer on the face in region of the inner corner of the eye or around the nose.

Roentgen, measure of radiation.

Roentgenogram, x-ray.

Rongeur, gouge forceps used to remove bone fragments.

Root, proximal end of a nerve; portion of an organ implanted in tissues.

Root Canal, pulp cavity of tooth root.

Rosacea, skin disease of the face in which there is permanent redness over the nose and cheeks.

Rose Fever, hay fever.

Roseola, red rash from various causes.

Rose Rash, any red colored eruption.

Rossbach's Disease, excessive secretion of gastric juice.

Rot, decay.

Rotate, twist; revolve.

Rotula, kneecap or patella.

Rotular, pertaining to the kneecap.

Roughage, coarse material.

Roundworm, an intestinal parasite.

Roust, delivery room nurse who carries out unsterile tasks.

Rubedo, temporary redness of skin.

Rubella, German measles.

Rubeola, measles.

Rubor, redness of skin due to infection.

Rubrum, red.

Ructus, belching.

Rudimentary, elementary; undeveloped.

Ruga, fold or crease.

Rugose, wrinkled.

Rule of Nine, a method of determining the extent of burns.

Rumination, regurgitation,

Rump, buttocks.

Run, to exude pus or mucus.

Runaround, infection extending around a finger or toenail.

Rupophobia, extreme dislike for dirt or filth.

Rupture, tearing apart; hernia.

Rutilizm, red-headedness.

Rx, symbol for "take" or "recipe."

Saburra, foulness of stomach or mouth.

Sac, pouch.

Saccharin, sugar substitute; sweetener.

Saccharum, sugar.

Sacculation, grouping of sacs.

Saccule, small sac.

Sacrificial Operation, removal of an organ for the patient's good.

Sacroiliac, relating to the juncture of the hipbone and lower part of the spine.

Sacroiliac Strain, type of backache.

Sacrum, part of vertebral column or spine.

Sadism, perversion in which sexual pleasure is obtained by inflicting pain on someone.

Sadist, one who enjoys inflicting pain on others.

St. Vitus' Dance, involuntary muscular action.

Sal, salt.

Salacious, lustful.

Salicylate, main component of aspirin.

Saline, pertaining to salt.

Saline Solution, salt water.

Saliva, fluid secreted by the glands of the mouth.

Salivant, stimulating secretion of saliva.

Salivary, pertaining to saliva.

Salivary Glands, three pairs of glands, located in the vicinity of the mouth, that secrete saliva.

Salivation, excess secretion of saliva.

Sallow, having a pale, yellowish complexion.

Sal Mirabile, purgative salt.

Salmonella, bacteria causing intestinal disorder.

Salmonellosis, infestation with Salmonella bacteria.

Salpingectomy, surgical removal of Fallopian tube.

Salpingitis, inflammation of the Fallopian tubes.

Salpinx, uterine tube; eustachian tube.

Salt, sodium chloride.

Saltation, dancing.

Saltatory, characterized by leaping or dancing.

Salt Free Diet, diet which allows no more than two grams of salt.

Saltpeter, postassium nitrate.

Salubrious, promoting good health.

Salutary, healthful; curative.

Salve, ointment.

Sanative, healing.

Sanatorium, place for preserving health or caring for a long term illness.

Sanatory, promoting health.

Sane, of sound mind.

Sanger's Operation, type of Cesarean section.

Sangucolous, inhabiting the blood.

Sanguifacient, forming blood.

Sanguiferous, conducting blood.

Sanguine, bloody.

Sanguineous, bloody; having a plethora of blood.

Sanguis, blood.

Sanitarium, place for the care and cure of those suffering from mental or physical illness.

Sanitary, pertaining to health.

Sanity, soundness of mind.

Saphena, large vein of leg.

Sapid, possessing flavor.

Sapo, soap.

Saponatus, mixed with soap.

Sapphism, lesbianism.

Sapremia, blood poisoning.

Saprodontis, tooth decay.

Sarcitis, inflammation of muscle tissue.

Sarcocele, tumor of testicle.

Sarcode, protoplasm.

Sarcogenic, forming flesh.

Sarcology, study of soft body tissues.

Sarcolytic, decomposing flesh.

Sarcoma, one of the two main types of cancer, the other being carcinoma.

Sarcophagy, practice of eating flesh.

Sarcopoietic, forming flesh or muscle.

Sarcous, pertaining to flesh or muscle.

Sartorius, muscle of thigh.

Satiety, satisfying fullness.

Saturated Fat, a fat so constituted chemically that it is not capable of absorbing any more hydrogen.

Saturnine, pertaining to lead.

Saturnism, lead poisoning.

Satyriasis, abnormal sex drive associated with mental excitement in male.

Satyromania, excessive sexual desire in the male.

Savory, appetizing.

Saw, cutting instrument.

Scab, crust formation over wound.

Scabies, disease of the skin caused by a mite which burrows under the skin surface and causes extreme discomfort and itching.

Scald, burn of skin.

Scale, small, thin, dry particle.

Scalenus, three muscles located in the vertebrae of the neck and attached to the first two ribs.

Scall, scalp disease.

Scalp, hairy component of head.

Scalpel, surgical knife.

Scanty, insufficient.

Scapula, shoulder blade.

Scapular, pertaining to the shoulder blade.

Scapulectomy, surgical removal of scapula.

Scar, end product of healed wound.

Scarfskin, epidermis.

Scarlatina, scarlet fever.

Scarlet Fever, contagious disease causing chills, high fever, sore throat, skin rash, discolored tongue.

Scatacratia, fecal incontinence.

Scatemia, intestinal toxemia.

Scatology, study and analysis of waste product of body.

Scelalgia, pain in leg.

Schick Test, test for susceptibility to diphtheria.

Schistasis, any congenital fissure.

Schizophrenia, psychiatric disorder of many and varied manifestations in which person loses contact or misinterprets reality.

Schizotrichia, splitting of hair.

Schwelle, threshold.

Sciage, sawing massage movement.

Sciatica, inflammation of or injury to the sciatic nerve in back of thigh.

Sciatic Nerve, largest nerve in body located in back of leg.

Scirrhoma, scirrhus.

Scirrhus, hard cancer.

Schlera, white of eye.

Schlerectomy, surgical removal of part of the sclera.

Schleritis, inflammation of the white of the eye.

Schleroderma, skin disease of unknown origin in which patches of skin become thickened, hard and white or yellowish.

Scleroma, sclerosis.

Sclerose, to become hardened.

Sclerosis, hardening of a tissue.

Sclerothrix, abnormal hardness and dryness of hair.

Scoliosis, curvature of the spine to one side or the other.

Scopophobia, extreme fear of being seen.

Scorbutus, scurvy.

Scordinemia, yawning and stretching.

Scotoma, blind spot.

Scotophobia, extreme fear of darkness.

Scotopia, adjustment of eyes to darkness.

Scours, diarrhea.

Scratch, superficial injury.

Scrobiculate, pitted.

Scrobiculus, pit.

Scrobiculus Cordis, pit of the stomach.

Scrofula, condition of tuberculous gland of the neck.

Scrotal, pertaining to the scrotum.

Scrotum, pouch of male containing testicles.

Scrub Nurse, operating room nurse.

Scruf, dandruff.

Scurvy, disease due to lack of vitamin C, causing bleeding, weakness and swelling of skin.

Scutum, thyroid cartilage.

Scytitis, dermatitis.

Sea Sickness, nausea, vomiting and unsteadiness due to unusual motion.

Sebaceous, pertaining to sebum.

Sebaceous Cyst, a wen; a swelling caused by the blocking of a duct of a sebaceous gland.

Sebaceous Glands, glands that are associated with the hair follicles. They secrete oil (sebum) into the hair follicles near the surfaces of the skin.

Sebastomania, religious insanity.

Seborrhagia, excessive secretion of sebaceous glands.

Seborrhea, condition of excessive oiliness of the skin caused by glandular upset.

Sebum, oily secretion of the oil glands of the skin.

Secondary, not of primary importance.

Secondary Hypertension, an elevated blood pressure that is caused by (and therefore secondary to) certain specific diseases or infections.

Secreta, waste material expelled by a gland or organ.

Secretin, a hormone produced in the small intestine. Secretin stimulates the pancreas and the liver.

Secretion, fluid discharged from gland or organ.

Secretomotory, stimulating secretion.

Section, divide by cutting.

Sectorial, cutting.

Secundigravida, woman in her second pregnancy.

Secundines, afterbirth material.

Sedative, agent used to quiet patient.

Sediment, material which settles at the bottom of a fluid.

Seed, semen.

Segment, part of a whole.

Seizure, sudden attack.

Sella, saddle-shaped depression; area within skull.

Semantic, pertaining to the meaning of words.

Semeiosis, approach to disease according to symptoms.

Semel, once.

Semen, male secretion containing sperm.

Semenuria, presence of semen in urine.

Semi- (prefix), half.

Semicircular Canals, three small tubes located in each ear.

Semilunar, wrist bone.

Seminal Vesicles, two pouches that are situated (in the male) between the bladder and the rectum. They secrete and store a fluid to be added to the secretion of the testes at the time of ejaculation.

Semination, introduction of semen into the vagina.

Seminiferous, producing or carrying semen.

Seminology, study of semen.

Semis, half.

Senescence, process of growing old.

Senile, old.

Senilism, premature old age.

Sensation, awareness of stimulus to nervous system.

Sense, perceive through nervous system; perceiving faculty.

Sensibility, sensitivity.

Sensitive, responsive; unusually receptive to stimuli.

Sensorium, any sensory nerve center.

Sensory, pertaining to sensation.

Sentient, sensitive.

Sepsis, poisoning of body by products of bacteria.

Septicemia, blood poisoning.

Septum, tissue dividing cavities.

Sequela, after affects of a disease.

Sequestrum, piece of dead bone.

Serial, arranged in sequence.

Seriate, saw-toothed.

Serology, study of serum.

Serosa, layer of tissue.

Serotonin, a naturally occurring compound that is found mainly in the gastrointestinal tract and in lesser amounts in the blood. Serotonin has a stimulating effect on the circulatory system.

Serous, thin and watery.

Serous Membrane, lining tissues of the body that are moistened by a fluid resembling the serum of the blood.

Serrate, notched.

Serrulate, minutely notched.

Serum, clear fluid which separates from blood when it clots.

Sesamoid Bone, a bone that develops within a tendon.

Sex, distinctive feature between male and female; Freud-pleasure.

Sex Hormones, the hormones that control and stimulate the growth of the secondary sex characteristics.

Sexual, pertaining to sex.

Shank, leg from knee to ankle.

Sheath, tubular case.

Shift, change.

Shigella, organism causing dysentery.

Shin, front part of lower leg.

Shingles, herpes zoster, viral infection of nerve path.

Shin Splints, a condition in which there is pain in the front of the lower part of the leg due to strained and swollen muscles, frequently caused by an excess of exercise or sports.

Ship-Fever, typhus fever.

Shiver, chill.

Shock, decreased effective circulating fluid volume.

Shortsighted, not able to see very far.

Shoulder, joint between arm and body.

Show, vaginal discharge prior to start of labor.

Shunt, a passage between two blood vessels or between the two sides of the heart where an opening exists in the wall that normally separates them.

Sialaden, salivary gland.

Sialadenitis, inflammation of a salivary gland.

Sialine, pertaining to saliva.

Sialism, increased production of saliva.

Sialogogue, causing the secretion of saliva.

Sialoporia, deficient saliva secretion.

Sialorrhea, flowing of saliva.

Sibilant, whistling; hissing.

Sibling, brother or sister.

Siccative, drying.

Sick, not in normal health.

Sickle Cell Anemia, a chronic disorder of the blood characterized by red blood cells that are sickle or crescent-shaped.

Sickness, illness.

Side Effect, an effect that is aside from or in addition to the desired effect. Side effects occur as a result of taking medicines or other kinds of treatments.

Siderodromophobia, extreme fear of train travel.

Sigh, involuntary inspiration of emotional origin.

Sight, act of seeing.

Sigmatism, faulty pronunciation of s sound.

Sign, symptom, evidence.

Signature, directions for taking medicine on a prescription.

Silicosis, condition of the lungs found in those who work among stone dust.

Sinapism, mustard plaster.

Sinciput, upper part of head.

Sinew, tendon or fibrous tissue.

Singultus, hiccough.

Sinister, left.

Sinistrad, toward the left.

Sinistral, pertaining to the left side.

Sinoatrial Node, a small mass of specialized cells in the right upper chamber of the heart that give rise to the electrical impulses that initiate contractions of the heart.

Sinuous, winding.

Sinus, hollow area of a bone.

Sinuses of Valsalva, three pouches in the wall of the aorta (the main artery leading from the left lower chamber of the heart) located behind the three cup-shaped membranes of the aortic valve.

Sinusitis, inflammation of the nasal sinuses.

Sinusotomy, incision of a sinus.

Sippy Diet, diets used to decrease acid or stomach juice.

Siriasis, sunstroke.

Sitology, study of food and its use.

Sitophobia, extreme dislike of food.

Situs, position.

Sitz-Bath, a therapeutic bath in sitting position.

Skelalgia, leg pain.

Skeleton, bones of body.

Skin, outer covering of body.

Skull, bones of head, 22 in all.

Sleep, normal loss of consciousness.

Sleeping Sickness, an infection of brain causing increased drowsiness; encephalitis.

Sling, support of arm or leg.

Slipped Disk, a vertebral disk that has slipped or been displaced.

Slough, dead tissue which separates from living tissue.

Smallpox, serious infectious disease with fever, pain, vomiting and an eruption of red spots which later become blisters and afterwards are filled with pus.

Smear, preparation of body secretions spread on a glass slide for microscopic study.

Smegma, thick, odorous secretion of certain glands.

Smog, mixture of smoke and fog.

Smell, odor; to stimulate olfactory cells.

Snakebite, the body's physical reaction to the venom injected by the bite of a snake.

Sneezing, a nose irritation which causes sudden expulsion of air from mouth and nose.

Snoring, a nose or throat obstruction causing a noise when breathing during sleep.

Snowblindness, temporary loss of sight due to glare on snow.

Snuffles, yellow discharges from nose of infants.

Soak, immerse in a solution.

Sociology, study of social relationships.

Socket, hollow into which another part fits.

Sodium, a mineral that is essential to life. It is found in nearly all plant and animal tissue.

Sodokosis, rat-bite fever.

Sodomy, unusual sexual relations, bestiality.

Soft, not hard or firm.

Soft Palate, posterior part of palate.

Solar, pertaining to the sun.

Solar Fever, infectious febrile disease.

Solar Plexus, anatomical area in upper part of abdomen.

Sole, bottom of foot.

Soleus, soft, broad muscle of calf or leg.

Solid, not hollow, gaseous or liquid.

Soluble, able to be dissolved.

Solute, substance which is dissolved in a solution.

Solution, homogeneous mixture of a solid in a liquid.

Solvent, solution used to dissolve material.

Soma, the body.

Somal, pertaining to the body.

Somatalgia, bodily pain.

Somatesthesia, bodily sensation.

Somatic, pertaining to the body.

Somnambulism, sleepwalking.

Somnifacient, causing sleep.

Somniferous, causing sleep.

Somniloquism, talking while asleep.

Somnolent, sleepy.

Soor, thrush.

Sophistication, adulteration of a product.

Sopor, coma.

Soporific, producing sleep.

Sore, an ulcer or wound.

Sore Throat, inflammation of pharynx, tonsils or larynx.

Sororiation, growth of breasts at puberty.

Soterocyte, blood platelet.

Sound, noise; auditory sensations caused by vibrations.

Space, area; region, segment.

Span, distance from fingertip to fingertip with arms outstretched.

Spanogyny, decrease in female births.

Spargosis, swelling of female breasts with milk; thickening of skin.

Spasm, contraction of any muscle that is sudden and involuntary.

Spasmodic, occurring in spasms.

Spasmophemia, stuttering.

Spasmophilia, tendency to spasms.

Spasmus, spasm.

Spastic, rigid; flexed; pertaining to spasms.

Spasticity, sustained increased muscle tension.

Spay, to remove female sex gland.

Specialists, one skilled in a particular field.

Species, category; classification.

Specimen, part of tissue or material used for analysis.

Spectacles, eye glasses.

Speculum, instrument which widens the opening of body cavities for examination.

Speech, thought expressed in words.

Sperm, male fertilizing cell.

Spermatocidal, killing sperm.

Sphacelate, to become gangrenous.

Sphacelation, gangrene.

Spheroma, spherelike tumor.

Sphincter, muscle that surrounds and closes an opening.

Sphincterismus, spasm of sphincter.

Sphygmic, pertaining to the pulse.

Sphygmomonometer, blood pressure gauge.

Spica, figure-of-8 bandage.

Spina, sharp protuberance; spine.

Spina Bifida, condition in which there is a defect in the development of the spinal column.

Spinal, pertaining to a spine.

Spinal Column, a series of bones in the back. The spinal column encloses and protects the spinal cord.

Spinal Cord, part of nervous system enclosed within the backbone; part of the nervous system which transmits impulses to and from the brain.

Spinal Curvature, condition where spine is abnormally bent forward or backward.

Spinal Fracture, broken back.

Spinal Nerves, the thirty-one pairs of nerves that start in the spinal cord and leave the spinal column through the spaces between the vertebrae.

Spine, sharp piece of bone; backbone.

Spinthecism, seeing sparks before the eyes.

Spirit, volatile liquid; alcoholic liquid.

Spirits of Ammonia, a fluid solution containing ammonia and alcohol.

Splanchnic, concerning abdominal organs.

Spleen, organ situated in the left upper part of the abdomen which manufactures, stores and destroys blood cells.

Splenalgia, pain in the spleen.

Splenauxe, enlargement of the spleen.

Splenectomy, surgical removal of spleen.

Splenic, pertaining to the spleen.

Splenitis, inflammation of the spleen.

Splenoma, splenic tumor.

Splenomegaly, enlargement of the spleen.

Splint, appliance to protect or stabilize injured part.

Spondyle, vertebra.

Spondylitis, inflammation of spine.

Sporadic, intermittent; occurring at different times and places.

Spot, blemish.

Sprain, injury of a joint caused by over-stretching of the ligaments.

Sprue, disease in which the patient is unable to absorb necessary nutrients.

Spur, pointed outgrowth.

Sputum, material that is spat out of mouth.

Squama, scale.

Squatting, sitting on the heels.

Stab, puncture with sharp object.

Stabilization, making firm and steady.

Stable, immobile.

Stactometer, device for measuring drops.

Staff, hospital personnel.

Stalagmometer, instrument for measuring drops.

Stamina, endurance.

Stammering, hesitant speech.

Stanch, to stop a flow of blood.

Stapedectomy, an operation to correct a hearing loss that has been caused by otosclerosis.

Stapes, small bone of middle ear.

Staphylococcus, bacteria causing body infection.

Staphyloma, budging of the white of the eye.

Starch, a form of carbohydrate.

Starvation, continued deprivation of food.

Stasis, stoppage of flow of blood or urine.

Stasophobia, extreme fear of standing up.

Stat., at once.

State, condition.

Statim, at once.

Status, condition; state.

Steatitis, inflammation of fatty tissue.

Steatopygia, having large buttocks.

Stillate, star-like shape.

Stenochoria, stenosis.

Stenosed, narrowed; constricted.

Stenosis, constricted; decrease in diameter.

Stercus, excrement.

Stereotypy, persistence of a single idea.

Sterile, barren; aseptic.

Sterility, inability to have children.

Sterilize, to make bacteria free; remove ability to reproduce.

Sterilizer, device for eliminating bacteria on instruments.

Sternal, pertaining to the sternum.

Sternalgia, pain in the sternum.

Sternodynia, pain in breastbone.

Sternum, breastbone.

Sternutation, sneezing.

Steroids, a collective term for a group of chemically similar compounds.

Stertor, snoring.

Stethalgia, chest pain.

Stethoscope, instrument used to listen to sounds of body.

Sthenia, force; strength.

Stigma, mark or spot on tissue.

Stigmatosis, skin disease characterized by ulcerated spots.

Stillbirth, birth of a dead baby.

Stillborn, born dead.

Stimulant, anything that increases activity.

Stimulus, exciting agent.

Stitch, localized sharp pain; sewing loop.

Stokes-Adams Syndrome, sudden attacks of unconsciousness.

Stoma, mouth.

Stomach, large pouch where food digestion begins.

Stomach Ulcers, sores or ulcer in stomach wall usually due to increased secretion of acid.

Stomachalgia, pain in the stomach.

Stomachic, gastric stimulant.

Stomatalgia, pain in mouth.

Stomatitis, inflammation of the mouth.

Stomatodynia, pain in mouth.

Stomatopathy, any mouth disorder.

Stool, feces.

Strabismus, squint, cross-eye.

Strain, overexertion; overstretching.

Strait, narrow passage.

Strangulation, choking; stopping of blood supply.

Strangury, painful urination.

Strap, bind with bandages.

Stratified, layered.

Stratum, layer of tissue nearly uniform in thickness.

Streak, line; stripe.

"Strep" Throat, a common childhood illness caused by a bacterial infection, which is treated with antibiotics.

Streptococcus, an organism infecting man.

Streptomycin, an antibiotic drug.

Stress, physical or emotional factor which causes tension in the body or in the mind. Stress is often a contributory factor in heart disease, ulcers, and elevated blood pressure, as well as other illnesses.

Stretcher, device for carrying the sick.

Stria, linear mark or line on body.

Striate, having streaks.

Stricture, narrowing of any tube in the body.

Stridor, harsh, rasping breath sound.

Stroke, apoplexy; seizure; fit.

Stroke Volume, the amount of blood that is pumped out of the heart at each contraction of the heart.

Stroma, framework of an organ.

Struma, goiter.

Strumectomy, thyroidectomy.

Strychnism, strychnine poisoning.

Stump, remaining part of limb after amputation.

Stun, momentary loss of consciousness.

Stupefacient, narcotic.

Stupemania, manic stupor.

Stupor, state of decreased feeling.

Stuttering, speech impediment characterized by repeating syllables.

Sty, infection of gland of eyelid.

Subacute, mildly acute.

Subclavian, below collar bone.

Subclavian Arteries, two large arteries that are located beneath the clavicle or shoulder bone.

Subconscious, out of awareness.

Subcostal, below a rib.

Subcutaneous, under the skin.

Subcutaneous Tissue, tissue located beneath the skin.

Subdelirium, mild delirium.

Sublatio, detachment of a part.

Sublimation, process of passing from solid to vapor state without liquifying.

Subliminal, below conscious awareness.

Sublingual Gland, salivary gland beneath tongue.

Subluxation, minor dislocation.

Submaxilla, mandible.

Submixillary Gland, salivary gland along jaw.

Submental, beneath the chin.

Subphrenic, beneath the diaphragm.

Subscription, part of a prescription giving directions for compounding the ingredients.

Substance, material of which a thing is composed.

Substantia, substance.

Subtotal, incomplete.

Sububeres, unweaned infants.

Subungual, beneath a nail.

Subvirile, lacking in virility.

Succorrhea, excessive secretion.

Succus, fluid secretion.

Sucrose, a complex sugar.

Sudation, perspiring.

Sudatorium, sweat bath.

Sudden Infant Death, the sudden, unexpected and unexplained death of an apparently healthy baby. This syndrome attacks infants between the ages of two weeks and two years.

Sudor, sweat.

Sudoresis, excessive sweating.

Suffocation, blockage of air ways.

Suffusion, spreading; diffusion.

Sugar, carbohydrate.

Suicide, self-destruction.

Sulcus, groove or furrow.

Sulfa Drugs, name referring to the group of drugs used in the treatment of various bacterial diseases.

Sulfonamides, a class of drugs used to treat infections that are caused by bacteria.

Sulfur, a pale-yellow, naturally occurring element used to treat infections or problems caused by fungus or by parasites.

Sunburn, skin inflammation from sun's rays.

Sunstroke, stroke due to excessive exposure to the sun.

Superalimentation, excessive feeding.

Superciliary, concerning eyebrow.

Supercilium, eyebrow.

Superego, conscience.

Superficial, near the surface.

Superinfection, an occasional complication that follows the use of antibiotics for the treatment of infections.

Superlactation, oversecretion of milk.

Supernumeray, more than usual.

Superscription, R͟x before a prescription.

Supinate, turn hand upward.

Supine, lying flat on back.

Suppository, solid medication for insertion into a cavity other than the mouth.

Suppurate, form infection.

Sura, calf of the leg.

Sural, pertaining to the calf.

Suralimentation, overfeeding.

Surditas, deafness.

Surdomute, deaf and dumb.

Surgeon, medical specialist performing surgery.

Surgery, specialty of medicine that deals with disease and trauma by operative means.

Surgical, pertaining to surgery.

Surrogate, a substitute.

Susceptible, having little resistance, easily influenced.

Suspiration, sigh.

Suspirious, breathing heavily.

Susurration, murmur.

Suture, to stitch together.

Swab, gauze wrapped around a stick for application of medicine.

Sweat, perspiration.

Sweat Gland, a coiled, tubular gland embedded in the dermis.

Syllepsis, pregnancy.

Symbiosis, a relationship between two organisms in which one organism harbors or nourishes another organism.

Symmetry, similar parts on opposite sides.

Sympathetic Nervous System, one of two parts of the autonomic nervous system. With the parasympathetic nervous system, the sympathetic nervous system regulates tissues not under voluntary control, such as the glands, the heart, and the smooth muscles.

Symphysis, immovable joint.

Symphysis Pubis, pubic bones above the midline of the external genital.

Symptom, perceptible change from normal function.

Syndrome, any group of symptoms commonly occurring together.

Synechia, abnormal joining of parts.

Synergists, drugs that work together. The combined effect of the drugs is greater than the normal effects of the separate drugs.

Synergy, cooperation.

Syngamy, sexual reproduction.

Synizesis, contraction of the eye pupil.

Synovial Membranes, membranes that serve as linings for joints.

Synovitis, inflammation of the lining of a joint.

Syntaxis, junction of two bones.

Syphilis, serious venereal disease.

Syrinx, cavity or tube.

Systemic Circulation, the circulation of the blood through all parts of the body except the lungs.

Systole, period during which contraction of heart takes place.

Tabefacation, emaciation.

Tabes, gradual deterioration in chronic illness.

Tabes Dorsalis, a disease of the nervous system leading to paralysis and caused by syphilis.

Tablet, pill.

Tabule, pill.

Tache, spot; blemish.

Tachycardia, rapid beating of the heart coming on in sudden attacks.

Tachylalia, rapid speech.

Tachyphagia, rapid eating.

Tachyphasia, rapid speech.

Tachypnea, unusually fast rate of breathing.

Tachyrhythmia, rapid heart action.

Tactile, pertaining to sense of touch.

Tactual, pertaining to touch.

Tactus, touch.

Taenia, band-like muscle or tissue; tapeworm.

Tagma, protoplasm.

Talalgia, pain in the heel.

Talc, a powder.

Talipes, club foot.

Talipes Planus, flatfoot.

Tallus, ankle.

Tampon, round cotton plug used to close wound or cavity.

Tamponade, act of plugging.

Tannic Acid, one of the most valuable astringents (drugs that have the power to contract tissue).

Tap, puncture of body cavity.

Tapeworm, type of intestinal worm.

Taphephobia, extreme fear of live burial.

Tarsal, pertaining to the eyelid or the instep.

Tarsus, arch of foot.

Tartar, dental calculus.

Taste, sensation through nerves on tongue.

T.A.T., toxin-antoxin.

Taxonomy, science of classification of plants and animals.

Tay-Sachs Disease, an inherited disorder that destroys the nervous system and is always fatal. Tay-Sachs disease is caused by the absence of an enzyme (called hexosaminidase) that normally aids in the breakdown of fat.

Tear, saline fluid secreted by lacrimal glands.

Teat, nipple.

Technic, technique.

Technique, method; procedure.

Tectonic, pertaining to plastic surgery.

Tectum, roof-like structure.

Teeth, bony growths in jaw used for chewing.

Teeth, Milk, first set of teeth.

Teething, appearance of teeth.

Tegmen, covering.

Tegument, skin.

Teinodynia, pain in the tendons.

Tela, weblike structure.

Telalgia, referred pain.

Telangitis, inflammation of capillaries.

Telangiosis, disease of capillary vessels.

Teleorganic, vital.

Telepathist, mind reader.

Telepathy, communication of two minds at a distance through means undetectable by science.

Telergy, automatism.

Telesthesia, extrasensory perception.

Temperament, physical and mental characteristics of an individual.

Temperature, degree of heat and cold; body temperature is normally 98.6.

Temple, area in front of ear.

Temporal, pertaining to the temple or time.

Temulence, drunkenness.

Tenacious, adhesive.

Tenalgia, pain in a tendon.

Tenderness, soreness.

Tendinitis, inflammation of a tendon.

Tendinous, pertaining to or composed of tendons.

Tendo, tendon.

Tendon, fibrous tissue that connects muscles to other structures.

Tenectomy, surgical removal of a tendon.

Tenesmus, spasm of anus or bladder.

Tenia, tapeworm; band.

Teniacide, medication which destroys tapeworms.

Tennis Elbow, pain in the arm, particularly on twisting inwards, caused by excessive strain.

Tenodynia, pain in a tendon.

Tenonitis, inflammation of tendon.

Tenoplasty, surgical repair of a tendon.

Tenorrhaphy, suture of a tendon.

Tenosynovitis, inflammation of a tendon and its sheath.

Tension, condition of being strained or stretched.

Tentative, subject to change.

Tentigo, unusual sex desires.

Tephrosis, cremation.

Tepid, warm.

Tepidorium, warm bath.

Teras, fetal monster.

Teratism, fetal monster.

Teratoid, monster.

Teratology, science dealing with monstrosities and malformations.

Tere, to rub.

Terebration, boring.

Teres, round; smooth.

Term, boundary; definite period of time.

Terminal, end.

Terracing, suturing in several rows.

Terror, extreme fear.

Testicles, the male reproductive glands.

Testis, male reproductive gland.

Tetanus, infectious disease characterized by painful spasms of voluntary muscles.

Tetany, disease characterized by painful muscle spasms with convulsive movements, usually due to inability to utilize calcium.

Tetracycline, a drug and a class of drugs that are antibiotics.

Tetralogy of Fallot, a congenital malformation of the heart involving four distinct defects.

Tetraplegia, paralysis of all four extremities.

Tetter, blister; pimple.

Textural, pertaining to the constitution of tissues.

Thalamus, area in the brain concerned with many bodily functions, often called the seat of the emotions.

Thalassemia, a disease resembling sickle-cell anemia.

Thalassophobia, extreme fear of sea.

Thalidomide, a sedative drug.

Thanatobiologic, pertaining to life and death.

Thanatoid, resembling death.

Thanatomania, suicidal obsession.

Thebaism, opium poisoning.

Theca, case; sheath.

Theism, poisoning from overdose of tea.

Thelalgia, pain in nipples.

Thelerethism, erection of the nipple.

Thelitis, inflammation of nipple.

Thelium, nipple.

Thenal, pertaining to the palm.

Thenar, area beneath thumb; palm.

Theomania, delusion that one is a deity.

Theory, hypothesis.

Therapeutic, pertaining to healing.

Therapeutics, scientific treatment of disease.

Therapist, a person skilled in the treatment of disease.

Therapy, treatment of disease.

Thermal, pertaining to heat.

Thermanalgesia, inability to react to heat.

Thermesthesia, perception of heat or cold.

Thermic, pertaining to heat.

Thermofuge, reducing fever.

Thermometer, instrument to measure heat.

Thermoplegia, heatstroke; sunstroke.

Thermostat, device for controlling heat.

Thigh, part of leg above knee.

Thiocyanate, a chemical that causes the dilation of the blood vessels, thus lowering blood pressure.

Thirst, desire for liquid.

Thoracalgia, chest pain.

Thoracic, pertaining to the chest.

Thoracectomy, surgical removal of a rib.

Thoracodynia, pain in thorax.

Thoracomyodynia, pain in chest muscles.

Thoracoschisis, fissure of chest wall.

Thoracotomy, surgical opening of chest.

Thorax, chest.

Threadworm, parasitic worm.

Threpsology, study of nutrition.

Threshold, point at which an effect is produced.

Thrill, heart murmur or abnormal blood vessel tremor that can be felt.

Thrix, hair.

Throat, area between mouth and esophagus.

Throb, pulsation.

Throe, sharp pain.

Thrombectomy, an operation to remove a blood clot from a blood vessel.

Thrombin, substance in blood which aids clotting.

Thrombocytes, blood platelets.

Thrombopathy, defective blood clotting.

Thrombophlebitis, inflammation of a vein.

Thrombosin, thrombin.

Thrombosis, formation of a clot within a blood vessel.

Thrombus, blood clot.

Thrush, disease of the mouth and throat caused by a fungus.

Thumb, first digit of hand.

Thymectomy, surgical removal of thymus.

Thymona, tumor of thyroid.

Thymion, wart.

Thymitis, inflammation of thyroid gland.

Thymona, tumor of thymus.

Thymus, glandular structure in the chest having an unknown function.

Thyroadenitis, inflammation of thyroid.

Thyrocele, goiter.

Thyrogenic, originating in thyroid.

Thyroid, glandular structure in the neck secreting thyroxin, a substance vital to life.

Thyroidectomy, surgical removal of all or part of the thyroid gland.

Thyroiditis, inflammation of the thyroid gland.

Thyrotropic Hormone, a hormone that influences the thyroid gland, stimulating the thyroid gland to secrete its hormone (thyroxin).

Thyroxin, hormone secreted by the thyroid gland.

Tibia, shin bone.

Tibial, pertaining to the tibia.

Tic, muscular twitch, usually of the face.

Tick, blood sucking parasite.

Tigroid, striped.

Tilmus, pulling out of hair.

Tincture, an alcoholic or hydroalcoholic solution used either for their therapeutic content or as flavoring agents or perfumes.

Tinea, ringworm.

Tinnitus, noises in the ear which may take the form of buzzing, clicking or thudding.

Tiqueur, one afflicted with a tic.

Tire, exhaust, fatigue.

Tissue, structure of body made up of similar cells.

Tissue Culture, the technique of growing plant or animal cells in containers outside the body by using a medium that contains a variety of nutrients.

Tobacosis, tobacco poisoning.

Tobagism, tobacco poisoning.

Tocalogy, obstetrical science.

Tocophobia, extreme fear of childbirth.

Tocus, childbirth.

Toe, digit of the foot.

Toilet Training, the method by which a child learns how to control his bowels and bladder.

Tolerance, endurance.

Tongue, organ of speech and taste.

Tongue-Tie, congenital shortening of frenuum below tongue.

Tonic, muscular tightness.

Tonometer, an instrument for measuring eye pressure.

Tonsil, mass or special lymph tissue.

Tonsilla, tonsil.

Tonsillectomy, removal of tonsils.

Tonsillitis, infection of the tonsils.

Tooth, hard structure in the jaws used for chewing.

Tophaceous, gritty, sandy.

Topical, pertaining to a particular spot.

Topoalgia, localized pain.

Toponarcosis, local anesthesia.

Torpidity, sluggishness.

Torpor, inactivity; apathy.

Torsion, twisting.

Torso, trunk of body.

Torticollis, wryneck; abnormal twisting of the neck caused by injury or infection to the muscle or nerve.

Torulus, small elevation.

Touch, tactile sense.

Tourniquet, band used to control bleeding.

Toxemia, any illness due to poisons absorbed from organisms in the system.

Toxenzyme, any poisonous enzyme.

Toxic, poisonous.

Toxicant, poisonous; a poison.

Toxicity, poisonous.

Toxicohemia, toxemia.

Toxicology, science dealing with poisons.

Toxicophobia, extreme fear of poisons.

Toxin, a term used to describe the poisonous substances released by bacteria.

Toxipathy, disease caused by poisoning.

T.P.R., temperature, pulse, respiration.

Trachea, the windpipe.

Tracheal, pertaining to trachea.

Tracheitis, inflammation of the windpipe.

Trachelagra, gout in the neck.

Trachelismus, spasm of neck muscles.

Tracheofissure, incision of trachea.

Tracheostomy, an emergency procedure to open the trachea and place a breathing tube through the opening down the trachea.

Tracheotomy, cutting into windpipe to relieve obstruction.

Trachitis, inflammation of trachea.

Trachoma, infectious disease of the eyes.

Trachyphonia, roughness of the voice.

Traction, pulling or drawing.

Tragopodia, knock-knee.

Trait, distinguishing characteristic.

Trance, sleeplike state.

Tranquilizer, calming agent.

Transcalent, able to be penetrated by heat rays.

Transfix, pierce.

Transforation, perforation of the skull of a fetus.

Transfusion, giving of one's blood to another.

Transmissable, communicable.

Transmission, communication of a disease from one person to another.

Transpirable, allowing passage of perspiration.

Transplant, remove tissue from one part of the body to another.

Transplantation, the removal of a body organ or body tissue from one individual and placing that organ or tissue in another individual.

Transverse, extending from side to side.

Transvestitism, uncontrollable urge to dress in the clothing of the opposite sex.

Trapizius, muscle of back.

Trauma, injury; wound.

Trauma, Psychic, injury to subconscious due to emotional shock.

Treatment, medical care of a patient.

Tremor, shake or quiver.

Tremulous, quivering.

Trench Mouth, mouth infection caused by organism; also called Vincent's angina.

Trend, course.

Trepan, to make a hole in skull to relieve pressure on brain.

Tresis, perforation.

Triamcinolone, a drug used in treating psoriasis.

Trichangiectasis, dilation of capillaries.

Trichauxe, excessive hair growth.

Trichinosis, disease caused by the trichina organism found in raw pork.

Trichitis, inflammation of the hair roots.

Trichobezar, hair-ball found in intestinal tract.

Trichocardia, hairy heart.

Trichoclasia, brittleness of hair.

Trichocryptosis, brittleness of hair.

Trichology, science of hair care.

Trichoptilosis, hair splitting.

Trichosis, any hair disease.

Tricuspid Valve, a valve consisting of three cusps or triangular segments; it is located between the upper and lower chamber in the right side of the heart.

Trifid, divided into three parts.

Trigeminal Nerve, one of the twelve pairs of cranial nerves.

Trigonid, first three cusps of a lower molar tooth.

Trilobate, having three lobes.

Triorchid, having three testes.

Triphasic, having three phases.

Triplegia, paralysis of three extremities.

Triplets, the birth of three babies as a result of a single pregnancy.

Triquetrum, wrist bone.

Trismus, spasm of jaw muscles.

Tristimania, melancholia.

Troche, lozenge.

Trochlear Nerve, one of the twelve pairs of cranial nerves.

Trochocardia, rotation of the heart on its axis.

Trochoides, pivot joint.

Trophic, pertaining to nutrition.

Trophic Nerves, specialized nerves that are concerned with the growth, nourishment, and repair of body tissues.

Trophology, science of body nutrition.

Trophonosis, any nutritional disease.

Truncal, pertaining to the trunk.

Truncate, cut off limbs or branches.

Truncus, trunk.

Trunk, torso.

Truss, device to hold hernia in place.

Trypsin, an enzyme produced by the pancreas.

Tube, long, hollow cylindrical structure.

Tuber, enlargement; swelling.

Tubercle, small swelling; rounded elevation on a bone; change in tissue caused by the tuberculosis germ.

Tuberculated, covered with tubercles.

Tuberculin, an extract made from dead tubercle bacilli (the cause of tuberculosis).

Tuberculophobia, extreme fear of tuberculosis.

Tuberculosis, infectious disease of man and animals caused by tubercle bacilli having many and varied manifestations in lungs, brain, bone, etc.

Tuberculous, caused by or having tuberculosis.

Tuberosity, bone projection.

Tubule, small tube.

Tuborrhea, discharge from eustachian tube.

Tularemia, an infectious disease transmitted by insects or small animals caused by the pasteurella organism.

Tumefaction, swelling.

Tumesence, swelling.

Tumor, a swelling or growth.

Tunic, lining membrane.

Tunnel, enclosed passage.

Turbidity, cloudiness.

Turgesence, distention; swelling.

Turgescent, becoming swollen.

Turgid, congested and swollen.

Turgor, swelling.

Tussis, cough.

Tutamen, a protection.

Twin, one of two persons of the same birth.

Twitch, slight muscular contraction.

Tyloma, callus.

Tylosis, formation of callosities.

Tympanal, pertaining to the tympanum.

Tympanic Membrane, a tightly stretched membrane that separates the auditory canal from the middle ear.

Tympanites, abdominal distention due to gas or air.

Tympanous, distended with gas.

Tympanum, ear drum.

Typhlosis, blindness.

Typhoid Fever, an infectious fever caused by the typhoid bacillus, characterized by diarrhea and other symptoms.

Typhomania, delirium found with typhoid fever.

Typhous, pertaining to typhus.

Typhus, a term indicating any one of a group of diseases and infections caused by rickettsia (a type of microorganism).

Uberous, prolific.

Uberty, fertility.

Ulalgia, pain in the gums.

Ulatrophia, shrinkage of gums.

Ulcer, sores on skin or internal parts of body caused by various things.

Ulceration, formation of an ulcer.

Ulcerative Colitis, an inflamed condition of the colon and rectum, which are the lowermost portions of the bowel.

Ulcus, ulcer.

Ulectomy, surgical removal of part of gums; removal of scar tissue.

Ulemorrhagia, bleeding from the gums.

Ulitis, gum inflammation.

Ulna, bone of forearm.

Ulnar, pertaining to the ulna.

Ulocace, ulcer and infection of gums.

Uloid, scarlike.

Ulorrhagia, bleeding from gums.

Ulosis, scar formation.

Ultrasound, diagnostic procedure using sound waves to produce a detailed image. Particularly valuable because it is neither painful nor harmful.

Ultraviolet Rays, invisible rays that are beyond the violet end of the spectrum.

Ululation, hysterical crying.

Umbilical Cord, the cord that connects the placenta at one end and the baby's navel at the other end.

Umbilicus, site on abdomen of attachment of umbilical cord.

Umbo, funnel-shaped area of ear drum.

Unciform, hook-shaped; bone of wrist.

Unconscious, state in which person is unaware of both his external and internal environment as in a faint.

Unction, ointment.

Unctuus, oily.

Undulant Fever, an infectious disease caused by the Brucella organism; found in animals and transmitted to man.

Undulation, wave.

Ungual, pertaining to the nails.

Unguent, ointment.

Unguis, fingernail or toenail.

Unilateral, pertaining to one side.

Unigravida, woman in her first pregnancy.

Union, juncture.

Unipara, woman who has borne one live child.

Universal Antidote, an antidote that has been devised for use when a patient has taken a poison but the exact nature or type of the poison is not known.

Uracratia, inability to retain urine.

Uraniscus, palate.

Uranium, radioactive element.

Urea, one of the waste products of the body's metabolic processes.

Uredo, sensation of burning on skin.

Uremia, poisoning from urinary substances in the blood.

Ureter, the tube leading from the kidneys to the bladder.

Ureterolith, stone in the ureter.

Uretha, tube which carries the urine from the bladder to the outside.

Urethritis, inflammation of the urethra.

Uretic, promoting urination.

Uric Acid, an organic substance that is a solid waste product contained in urine.

Urinary, pertaining to urine.

Urinary Meatus, the external opening of the male urethra located in the penis.

Urinate, discharge urine.

Urine, fluid end product of kidney activity.

Urologist, medical specialist who deals with organs producing and transportating urine.

Urology, study of the urinary systen

Uroschesis, to retain urine.

Urous, urine-like.

Urticaria, hives.

Ustion, incinerate, burn.

Ustus, burned.

Uterine, pertaining to the womb.

Uterus, womb.

Utricle, one of two small sacs located next to the cochlea of the inner ear.

Uvea, tissue layer of eye.

Uvula, small tissue projecting in the middle of palate in throat.

Vaccination, injection with a germ or germ product to produce immunity and protect against disease.

Vaccine, substance used for inoculation.

Vaccinia, contagious disease as a result of inoculation with cowpox virus.

Vagina, the passage connecting the outer and inner female sex organs.

Vaginismus, painful spasm of the vagina.

Vaginitis, inflammation of vagina.

Vagus, tenth cranial nerve.

Valence, ability of a chemical agent to combine in a reaction.

Valetudinarian, person afflicted with frequent illness.

Valgus, bowlegged; knock-kneed.

Valve, structure which prevents backward flow in a passage.

Valvular Insufficiency, a term applied to valves that close improperly and admit a backflow of blood in the wrong direction.

Valvulitis, inflammation of a valve.

Valvulotomy, incision of a heart valve.

Vaporizer, a small piece of equipment that heats water and releases it into the air.

Varicella, chickenpox.

Varices, enlarged, tortuoris vein.

Varicocle, varicose veins in the area of scrotum.

Varicose Veins, swollen veins caused by improper valve function.

Varicosities, an alternate term for varicose veins.

Variola, smallpox.

Vas, vessel, passageway.

Vascular, pertaining to blood vessels.

Vas Deferens, duct in testis which transports semen.

Vasectomy, excision of vas deferens; operation to sterilize male.

Vasoconstrictor, causing a narrowing of blood vessels.

Vasodepressor, agent which relaxes the blood vessels, thus increasing diameter and lowering blood pressure.

Vasodilator, an agent or substance that causes the blood vessels to relax.

Vasospasm, sudden decrease in caliber of blood vessel.

Vasopressor, a chemical substance that causes the muscles of the arterioles to contract, thus narrowing the arteriole passage and raising the blood pressure.

Vein, blood vessels carrying blood to heart.

Vena Cava, two large veins that empty into the heart.

Venereal, pertaining to sexual intercourse.

Venereal Disease, any infectious disease that is transmitted almost exclusively from person to person through sexual intercourse.

Venery, sexual intercourse.

Venesection, puncture of a vein to remove blood.

Venipuncture, surgical puncture of a vein.

Venom, poison from an animal.

Venous Blood, unoxygenated blood.

Ventricle, small cavity; pouch.

Ventricular Septum, the muscular wall that divides the left and right lower chambers of the heart (the ventricles).

Veratrum, a drug that lowers the blood pressure and decreases the heart rate.

Vermis, worm.

Vernix, a white, creamy substance that forms on the body of a fetus at about the seventh month.

Verruca, wart.

Version, turning; changing the position of the fetus in the womb to facilitate birth.

Vertebra, bone of the spinal column.

Vertex, crown of the head.

Vertical, pertaining to the vertex.

Vertigo, dizziness.

Vesica, bladder.

Vesicant, blistering.

Vesicle, blister; small bladder.

Vessel, tube; passageway.

Vestigial, non-functioning part in body more highly developed in embryo or lower animal.

Viable, alive.

Vibex, linear spots beneath skin due to hemorrhage.

Vibrissal, stiff hairs in nose.

Vibrio, a class of bacteria.

Vicious, faulty.

Vigil, wakefullness.

Villi, the minute, hairlike projections that cover the mucous membrane lining of the small intestine.

Vincent's Angina, mouth infection; also called trench mouth.

Vinum, wine.

Virgin, one who has not experienced sexual relations.

Virile, masculine, mature.

Virilism, maleness.

Virology, study of virus and viral diseases.

Virose, poisonous.

Virulence, poisonousness; infectiousness; endangering life.

Viruses, minute organisms which cause certain diseases among which are the common cold, measles, mumps, poliomyelitis, chickenpox, smallpox.

Vis, energy, power.

Viscera, organs within body.

Visceral Pericardium, the outer layer of the heart wall.

Viscid, thick; adherent.

Vision, sight; seeing.

Visual Field, the total area perceived when the eyes are focused straight ahead.

Vitals, important body organs.

Vital Signs, the temperature, pulse, and respiration of a patient.

Vitamins, chemical substances found in foods that are necessary for proper bodily function.

Vitiligo, lack of pigment in certain areas of the skin.

Vitium, a defect.

Vitiation, injury; decrease in function of a part.

Vitreous Body, the semifluid, transparent substance that lies between the retina and the lens of the eye.

Vivisect, to cut or dissect living animal.

Vocal Cords, tissue bands whose vibration causes speech.

Voice, sounds produced by the vibration of the vocal cords.

Void, to empty bladder or rectum.

Volce, palm or sole of foot.

Volition, act of selecting.

Volkmann's Contracture, a condition in which the fingers contract.

Volvulus, twisting of the bowel causing obstruction.

Vomer, bone of nose.

Vomicose, containing ulcers.

Vomiting, dislodging the food in stomach through mouth.

Vomitus, vomited material.

Vox, voice.

Voyeur, person receiving sexual pleasure from watching activities of others.

Vril, inborn energy from birth leading to maturity.

Vulva, female genital.

Vulvitis, inflammation of the female external genitalia.

Vulnus, wound.

—W—

Waist, area between chest and hip encircling body.

Walleye, a form of strabismus. Walleye is a condition in which one or both eyes turn out (as opposed to crossed eyes, in which the eyes turn in).

Wangensteen Tube, a tube that is inserted into the stomach through the nostrils and pharynx to provide constant drainage of the gastrointestinal tract.

Wart, growth on the skin that may be cause by viruses.

Wasserman Test, test of the blood to determine if syphilis is present.

Waste Products, substances that have entered the body (usually as food or beverages) but which cannot be used by the body and are excreted in the form of feces, urine, and sweat.

Water on the Knee, a condition in which there is an inflammation of the membrane in the knees. Fluid collects in the area as part of the inflammation.

Wean, substitution of other substances for breast milk.

Webbed, connected by a thin membrane.

Weeping crying; seeping of a fluid.

Wen, a sebaceous cyst.

Wernicke's Center, an area of the cerebral cortex of the brain. Wernicke's center is responsible for the ability to understand words that are spoken.

Wheal, a red, round elevation on skin.

Wheeze, sound in chest due to abnormalities in lungs.

Whiplash, injury to the neck sustained in a car accident in which the car is hit from behind, causing the neck to snap back and then forwards.

White Blood Cells, cells that allow the body to defend itself against disease.

White Leg, swelling and blanching of the leg produced by thrombosis of the veins.

Whooping Cough, infectious disease characterized by episodes of coughing punctuated by whooping noises between episodes during periods of gasping for breath, pertussis.

Wintergreen Oil, a salve or liniment used in the treatment of strained muscles and for relief of rheumatoid conditions.

Wisdom Tooth, the most posterior teeth or molar on each side of jaw.

Withdrawal Sickness, a term used to describe the various symptoms a drug or narcotics addict experiences when the use of the addicting substance is stopped abruptly.

Woman, mature female.

Womb, uterus; organ in which developing fetus resides.

Work Classification Unit, a community facility involving a team approach to assessing the ability of a cardiac patient to work in terms of the energy requirements of the job.

Wound, an injury or break in the skin.

Wrist, joint between forearm and hand.

Wryneck, torticollis; a condition that causes the head to turn to one side in spasms.

Xanthic, yellow.

Xanthocyanopsia, a form of color blindness in which the patient cannot tell the difference between green and red colors.

Xanthoma, yellow tumor or growth.

Xanthopsia, yellow vision.

Xanthosis, jaundice.

X Chromosome, one of the two sex chromosomes.

Xenogenous, disease caused by foreign body or toxin.

Xenomenia, bleeding from other than normal site at time of menstrual period.

Xenophobia, extreme fear of strangers.

Xenopthalmia, inflammation of eye due to foreign body.

Xeransis, condition of dryness.

Xerasia, dryness of hair leading to baldness.

Xerocheilia, dry lips.

Xeroderma, a skin disease characterized by dryness.

Xerophthalmia, eye condition in which the lining membrane of the lid and eyeball is dry and thickened.

Xerosis, condition of dryness.

Xerostomia, dryness of the mouth.

Xiphoid, sword-shaped cartilage at lowest part of breast bone.

X-Ray, device used to photograph interior parts of body; also used as therapeutic tool.

Xylometazoline, a drug used as a nasal decongestant.

Xysma, membranous like material in some diarrhea stools.

Xyster, surgical instrument used to scrape bone.

— Y —

Yawn, involuntary opening mouth when fatigued.

Yaws, tropical disease.

Y Chromosome, one of the two sex chromosomes.

Yeast, a rich source of vitamin B.

Yellow Bone Marrow, ordinary bone marrow in which fat cells predominate.

Yellow Fever, infectious fever found in tropical lands.

Yellow Mercuric Oxide, an ointment used as an antiseptic in the treatment of eye infections and in certain other skin infections where antibiotics cannot be used because of sensitivity.

Youth, period of adolescence between childhood and adult life.

— Z —

Zein, protein from corn.

Zestocausis, to burn with steam.

Zinc, a metal used in medicines.

Zoanthropy, belief that one is an animal.

Zoetic, pertaining to life.

Zondal-Aschheim Test, test to determine pregnancy.

Zonesthesia, sensation of tightness around the waist.

Zooerastea, coitus with an animal.

Zooid, animal-like.

Zoonoses, diseases of animals that accidentally affect man.

Zoopsia, hallucinations involving animals.

Zoosis, disease in man carried by animals.

Zoxazolamine, a drug that is used as a skeletal muscle relaxant.

Zygoma, a part of the cheek bone.

Zygote, a fertilized ovum, formed by the union of a sperm and an ovum.

Zyme, fermenting substance.